Ordinary Miracles

IN NURSING

Patricia Winstead-Fry, PhD, RN
CAM Nursing Research
Professor Emerita, University of Vermont
&
Deborah R. Labovitz, PhD, OTR/L, FAOTA
Professor of Occupational Therapy
The Steinhardt School of Education
New York University

JONES AND BARTLETT PUBLISHERS
Sudbury, Massachusetts
BOSTON   TORONTO   LONDON   SINGAPORE

World Headquarters
Jones and Bartlett
  Publishers
40 Tall Pine Drive
Sudbury, MA 01776
978-443-5000
info@jbpub.com
www.jbpub.com

Jones and Bartlett
  Publishers Canada
6339 Ormindale Way
Mississauga, Ontario L5V
1J2
CANADA

Jones and Bartlett
  Publishers International
Barb House, Barb Mews
London W6 7PA
UK

Jones and Bartlett's books and products are available through most bookstores
and online booksellers. To contact Jones and Bartlett Publishers directly, call
00-832-0034, fax 978-443-8000, or visit our website, www.jbpub.com.

Substantial discounts on bulk quantities of Jones and Bartlett's publications are
available to corporations, professional associations, and other qualified organizations. For details and specific discount information, contact the special sales department at Jones and Bartlett via the above contact information or send an email
to specialsales@jbpub.com.

ISBN-13: 978-0-7637-3814-3
ISBN-10: 0-7637-3814-X

Library of Congress Cataloging-in-Publication Data
Winstead-Fry, Patricia.
  Ordinary miracles in nursing / Patricia Winstead-Fry and Deborah R. Labovitz.— 1st
Jones and Bartlett ed.
    p. cm.
  ISBN 0-7637-3814-X
  1. Nursing—Anecdotes. I. Labovitz, Deborah. II. Title.
  RT82.W56 2006
  610.73—dc22
  6048   2005017230

Production Credits
Acquisitions Editor: Kevin Sullivan
Production Director: Amy Rose
Associate Editor: Amy Sibley
Marketing Manager: Emily Ekle
Manufacturing Buyer: Amy Bacus
Composition: Northeast Compositors
Cover Design: Timothy Dziewit
Printing and Binding: Malloy, Inc.
Cover Printing: Malloy, Inc.

Printed in the United States of America
10 09 08 07 06   10 9 8 7 6 5 4 3 2

DEDICATION

*This book is dedicated to all nurses whose stories, if they were known,
would be as compelling as those in this book.*

*It is also dedicated to the memory of the late Gail Fidler who was
Deborah's mentor and friend and to Susan Bachner, a true friend.*

CONTENTS

PREFACE

PATRICIA WINSTEAD-FRY, PHD, RN

DEBORAH R. LABOVITZ, PHD, OTR/L, FAOTA

As this book publishes, the United States health care system is the subject of debate between the two major political parties. Medicare is in its death throes, according to some. For others, it just needs some fine tuning. Private health insurance is getting more expensive and many Americans have no health insurance at all. In the midst of health care hubbub, hospitals and other organizations merge to create super-sized entities. Financial concerns dominate planning and decision making within these organizations. No good solution has emerged, as costs keep rising and consumer dissatisfaction with healthcare services increases.

Today, the United States is in the midst of a major nursing shortage. Such shortages have happened before but have not lasted as long or seemed as dire as today's. Many health care entities report a 20% vacancy of budgeted nursing positions. The causes of this shortage are many and not easily corrected. Among insurance company demands, managed-care demands, and health care systems managed only from a business perspective, acts that nurses value such as teaching patients about their illnesses and providing emotional support are not reimbursable. Therefore, these things are not done or are done at the risk of reprimand. Nurses can also make more money in other fields; so some leave.

Nurses work in stressful environments, often working mandatory double shifts (16 hours). The values of nursing are often seriously challenged, as the healthcare system wants to only treat the current episode of an illness. The idea that the patient may need other resources to prevent another episode is often not considered today. Patients and nurses, however, value positive outcomes and so do insurance companies. The values of prevention and health promotion are not totally lost in today's world, just harder to implement.

Yet people get sick, get pregnant, and are in accidents, creating new patients daily. Perhaps the most salient statement one can make about patients is that no one ever plans to be one. There are a few hypochondriacs who love medical diagnoses. For most people, however, a diagnosis is a traumatic, frightening event. Once one becomes a patient, the person enters a whole new world. The language is foreign. Invasive procedures may occur. Drugs and treatments, all with side effects, are prescribed. With a serious diagnosis, one's world turns upside down. With a less serious diagnosis, one learns new ways to navigate through life.

Wherever patients are, there are nurses. The nurse who works in a doctor's office may be the first healthcare professional one meets, as she takes blood pressure, temperature, and respirations. She may begin questioning about the onset and length of the symptoms that brought the patient to the doctor's office or clinic. Other nurses will be a part of treatment, case management, and home care.

Nurses and patients are entwined with one another. In a hospital setting, the nursing staff creates the environment the patient and family live within. In home care situations, the nurse visits patients and families in their home, often becoming part of the family. The stories in this book—some funny, some sad—are all real examples of the dynamics that occur between patients and nurses.

INTRODUCTION

PATRICIA WINSTEAD-FRY, PhD, RN

DEBORAH R. LABOVITZ, PhD, OTR/L, FAOTA

The stories in this book are about ordinary miracles that occur when patients and nurses come together. There is no rising of the dead, but a few deaths are averted because of the nurses' actions. There are heroic patients who survive and even flourish in the midst of serious medical conditions, supported by family and a nurse. The stories are miraculous because they show the depth of the human spirit. Whether the patient is in jail, an intensive care unit, or his own bed at home, when a nurse and a patient come together, there is the potential for magic.

For those readers whose impression of nurses is formed by television and movies, you will meet real nurses, who come in all shapes and sizes with good minds. Readers might be surprised by nurse practitioners who diagnose and prescribe. Nurses in intensive care units routinely perform ordinary miracles as they monitor patients, keeping them in balance so that wounds can heal or prematurity overcome. Nurses work creatively with the mentally challenged such as Elaine, the 63-year-old Downs Syndrome patient, who had serious heart disease. Elaine did not want oxygen, but she needed it. The nurse's creativity in explaining the consequences of removing oxygen is very impressive.

Patients can be demanding and downright nasty. Some are just that way, but others get dragged down by constant pain and loss of control over their lives. Helping patients recover some control and sense that they are managing the disease and not the other way around, unites patients and nurses in seeking a common goal. Whether it is having a daughter bring an elderly man's small poodle to visit him in the nursing home or procuring Matzoh for Passover for an inmate, nurses do the ordinary things that make life better, regardless of the setting.

Psychiatric patients can be dangerous to themselves and frightening to their families and to the nurses in the emergency department. One of the best and worst aspects of working in an emergency situation is that the nurse never knows who will be brought through the door. A young person hallucinating from drug use has to be cared for, even if he is spitting and swearing. Nurses who work in these situations have developed negotiating skills and creative solutions that are not covered in any standard textbook. Nurses who love emergency rooms are some of the most flexible, creative people in the world.

Infants and children with long-term illnesses are special patients who are seen throughout their lives by nurses. The patient, his family, and the nurses often spend long days and nights at the bedside. Strong bonds can be formed in these situations. This book has some special stories from school nurses who have a chance to influence children with lessons in what makes a good day. While all nurses assess patients, one's detective work in finding who had an intestinal parasite is worthy of a Perry Mason episode. It is never dull in the school nurse's office.

Nurses are everywhere. The section "Nurses in Unique Situations" contains stories from the current war in Iraq. A nurse who works with Holocaust survivors tells their story. Nurses who educate the next generation share incidents, including students' bravery on 9-11-01. One of the newest nursing specialties, Parish Nursing, is also represented. Parish Nursing was started about a decade ago by a Lutheran Pastor in the Chicago area, Rev. Granger Westberg. It is now recognized by the American Nurses Association and has its own standards of practice. Stories from staff development, occupational health and other advanced areas of practice are told. This section also contains stories of nurses as patients. Nurses, like everyone else, often get diagnoses that surprise and frighten them. Others, like Amy Heddon, who was stuck by a needle used to give medication to an HIV-positive child, avoided a devastating diagnosis.

Then there are stories of nurses as people, as they cope with taking care of elderly parents and sick children. A patient who challenges her nurse to pursue further education demonstrates the kind of mutual support that can evolve in nursing. Sometimes a party can be a source of educating the public about what nurses do, as Patrice Rancour shares.

Florence Nightingale described nurses as people who put patients in the best situation for nature to heal them. What constitutes healing varies with the patient's desires and the nurse's abilities to think and plan to meet the patient's needs. In one story a couple is in a car accident. The wife is badly hurt, the husband less so. When they bring the husband to see his wife in the emergency room, the couple begins to talk about a youngster who was also in the car. The nurses find out it is a puppy. They track down the pup at a fire station.

One of the nurses has her son pick up the puppy who has had no veterinarian care. The nurses notice that his hind leg is weak and get it x-rayed. That is total family-centered care.

Sometimes healing is a very active process of finding resources—both technical and personal—to get a patient moving in a positive direction. Such resources can include community programs for the homeless, a discharge plan that involves insurance carriers, the patient's employer, and the health care organization. Building teams that get patients in the best situation for them is a challenge, and when it works, it helps facilitate ordinary miracles.

CHAPTER 1

SPECIAL DELIVERY

BY KENDRA L. SMITH

The mom arrives on the obstetric unit at about 6 am. She is nervous and scared of the work ahead as she paces around the room continuously chattering. I ask the assessment questions while she paces around the room. I take her blood pressure, temperature, and respirations with her standing at the bedside. Thank goodness she stands still long enough for me to apply the fetal monitor. The baby is just fine. The final thing I need to do is check how dilated her cervix is, but the mom says she doesn't want to get into bed. I offer to check her while she is standing but explain that I can be more accurate if she is lying down. I promise her I will be as quick as possible. She looks so scared. She knows if she gets into the bed, she will have to have this baby. She decides to be in the bed, "but just for 5 minutes." It doesn't take long to discover that she is dilated to 4 centimeters and 100% effaced. She flies out of the bed and paces as far as the length of cord from the fetal monitor allows. She reminds me that she went from 4 to 10cm in 20 minutes with her first baby.

I call the doctor, give him the important information, and remind him she delivers quickly. Then I set up the room for the delivery. Just as I finish, the mom says she needs to empty her bladder. I unhook the monitor and she dashes to the bathroom. When she returns, she begins to do the ballerina move where she alternates her feet and goes up on the ball of her foot. This is a classic sign of rapid cervical dilation.

I ask the mom if I can check her again but she refuses. So, I ask her to let me know when she feels like pushing. I phone the doctor and he is in the shower. I call the emergency room for a doctor to come up to deliver the baby. The nursery nurse and I are informed that he is involved in a trauma case and is not available. We are on our own now.

We try again to get her into bed for the delivery. She is full of reasons not to. I point out to her that it is easier to guide the baby out if she is in bed, but I will do whatever she wants. With one more contraction, "the look" flashes across her face. All obstetric nurses know "the look." It is that realization that the baby is coming whether the mom is ready or not. She asks if the doctor is going to make it. I reassure her that he was called and should be here shortly. I also tell the mom that we never make a mom wait to deliver until her doctor is here. I think the mom knows the doctor is not going to make it.

She relents and hops into bed. (Yes, she really did hop!) The mom tells me, "the baby is coming." I tell her we are ready. As the baby descends she continues with her chatter, talking about anything and everything. The baby's head is emerging and I ask her if she would like to touch the baby's head. The mom says, "Yes," "No," "Yes." She tentatively places her fingers over her perineum. There are 7 centimeters of head right there. Her fingers spread apart to touch herself and the baby, trying to figure out where she ends and the baby begins. She realizes the baby will soon be here. "Oh it hurts so bad," she says. I ask her to drop her knees to the outside to decrease the pain. "It will hurt more," the mom says, and I answer back "No, it will get easier." Slowly she drops her knees to the outside and the relief is visible on her face. I tell her, "let the baby fill your hand." As she relaxes, the baby's head is delivered; she is caressing her infant's head.

As I support the baby's head while the delivery continues, I ask her if she wants to help me deliver her baby. She responds anxiously, "Is that what I came here for? Am I supposed to do that?" I simply state that she can help if she wants. She reaches down with a hand on each side of the baby's head. One shoulder delivers and then the other. As her baby glides from her body, her fingers are always touching the baby. As the baby's arms come free from her body, I help her put her hands under the baby's arms. She then lifts the baby free of her body, cradling her baby girl on her chest. The mom cries, "I did it, I did it, I did it." The baby is crying a lusty cry. The dad who has stood very quietly at the bedside the whole time is crying also. The baby's birth time was 6:37 am. The doctor arrived at 6:40 am.

The day shift comes on to assume care, giving me a chance to start and finish my paperwork. By the time I have completed and signed everything, the mom and baby are in the postpartum room. The baby is enjoying her first meal at the breast, while the mom eats a rather large breakfast as she talks on the phone to her family. I stop in to see her for just a minute, promising to see her again that night. She is still chattering away on the telephone. I don't think she stopped talking since she got here at 6:00 am.

When I return to work that night, the staff encourages me to go right into her room. She is quietly resting on her side. She tells me she hasn't slept all day. She has been on an emotional high since the baby was born. And then she says, "Can I ask you a question?" I say yes. I think I know what is coming. She asks, "If the doctor had been there, could I have touched my baby before she was born?" I answer, "Maybe." Her next question is: "Could I have delivered my own baby if the doctor had been there?" This time I shake my head in the negative. A mischievous grin appears on her face, and she says, "I am so glad he missed the delivery."

CHAPTER 2

THE CARDIAC BABY

BY CARRIE A. MOORE

It was supposed to be a routine admission. She was a baby girl named Sarah, born by Caesarean section. There were no known risk factors. I glanced at the clock as I put my stethoscope to her chest—9:30 pm. I was shocked as I listened to her heart sounds and heard the loudest murmur I have ever heard. I wanted a second opinion and called my partner, Lyn, over to listen. Her expression mirrored my reaction. We decided to check Sarah's oxygen saturation level because, in addition to the murmur, her skin color was unusual. Her oxygen level was dropping into the mid-eighties. We started giving her oxygen, which only improved her oxygen level minimally. In spite of the oxygen level, she did not appear to be in any respiratory distress. She was not grunting or having retractions or nasal flaring. Her lung sounds were clear. This was not typical for a C-section baby who is transitioning to extra-uterine life. We suspected that the problem was cardiac, not respiratory. I called her doctor who was not alarmed and he told me to keep monitoring her.

Fifteen minutes later her condition had not improved, so I put in another page to the pediatrician. When I could not reach him, Lyn and I decided to call Neonatal ICU (NICU) to see if there was someone who could come and take a look at Sarah. We were determined that a doctor would see this baby. In the meantime, Lyn kept administering oxygen and I obtained four extremity blood pressures which were a little abnormal but not alarmingly so. The NICU resident came over and ordered some labs and a chest x-ray (CXR). Sarah's primary pediatrician called back and talked to the NICU resident. He stated that he was on his way and he requested us to place Sarah under an oxyhood. These orders were carried out. All the results came back normal, except the

CXR report was delayed. After examining Sarah, the doctor was not unduly alarmed, stating the baby was just "transitioning." He walked over to the NICU to check the CXR results. A couple minutes later, he called back and told us Sarah would be transferred to NICU, and they would call us when they were ready for her.

What seemed like hours passed as Lyn and I waited for a call from the NICU. Lyn and I were taking turns monitoring her. Fifteen minutes later, NICU called to tell us that they were ready for the "cardiac baby." We were placing Sarah into the transporter as the NICU attending physician came over to check her. He listened to her heart sounds. He told us the CXR was abnormal and they were going to do an echocardiogram as soon as we transported her. We could not get there fast enough.

Once Sarah was safely in the NICU, Lyn and I returned to the newborn nursery and let out a sigh of relief. I glanced at the clock again. It was 1:00 am. An hour later, Sarah's pediatrician came back to the nursery. I asked him what was wrong with Sarah. He replied, "She has pulmonary stenosis. The murmur you heard was the ductus; it hadn't closed yet. If it had closed while she was here, she would have died. It's a good thing you called me about this."

Lyn and I looked at each other, speechless. The ductus arteriosis is a blood vessel that usually closes as soon as a baby takes her first cry; sometimes it can take a few hours to close after the baby is born. Sarah was born at 9:08 pm; she came to the nursery at 9:30 pm; we transferred her to NICU at 1:00 am. Four hours. The murmur we were so worried about was the one thing keeping her alive.

Sarah was transferred to another facility the next day where she eventually underwent open-heart surgery. The last we heard, she was home and recovering well. Lyn and I both praise God for keeping this precious child alive while she was under our care. And whenever anyone starts sharing memorable moments they have experienced in nursing, Lyn and I look at each other, smile, and remember Sarah.

CHAPTER 3

LAUNCHING OF A MIRACLE

By Pamela Daley LaFrentz

More years ago than I like to admit, I learned to deliver babies. It was part of the obstetrics rotation in our nursing program. Every time a baby was about to be born, our clinical instructor would hustle the student nurses who were on duty out of the labor room and into the delivery room with a smile and a wink and words of wonder: "The stork is flying low." By the end of our three-month rotation, we knew that every baby born was truly a launching of a miracle.

A short time after becoming an RN, I worked as a pediatric nurse in a small community hospital. The hospital designated less than ten pediatric beds, tucked away in an area that was once a sun porch off an adult medical surgical unit. On that sultry August morning, I was trying to deal with 6-year-old twins admitted pre-operatively for tonsillectomies, a baby with severe diarrhea, a kid with multiple broken body parts (car accident), and a box fan that sat in an ancient window, attempting to suck the hot air out of the unit, onto the hot asphalt below. In the midst of it all, Baby X arrived in a wet cloth diaper and a remarkably clean receiving blanket. He was one day old and unfit for the newborn nursery because he had been born outside the hospital. Healthy and perfect in every way, he was missing a mom and dad.

Once found, the infant was well protected: a parish priest, a police officer, and a social worker brought Baby X into my unit. At the time, I felt like I was playing a part in a Dickens novel. Here I was receiving a darling little baby boy who had been left on the doorstep of the rectory of the local Catholic Church while multiple social service agencies were trying to solve the mystery of his birth.

I remember asking the social worker as he handed the baby to me, "Why would anyone give up such a beautiful baby?" Even having trained at a large metropolitan teaching hospital, I had been shielded from many of life's harsh realities that some families and young people endure. On that day, the miracle of birth and the sorrowful realization of baby abandonment clashed forces. Over the years, of course, I have learned that babies are discarded in every town and every strata of society. I have no idea what the statistics on baby abandonment were in the United States in the early 1970s. I don't think the state or federal government was even tracking such statistics.

Nonetheless, on that distant summer morning, a pediatrician immediately examined Baby X and found no problems with him: ten fingers, ten toes, and ten feedings a day. He was born hungry and he let us know it. The nurse aide who worked with me in pediatrics would have absconded with the infant in a heartbeat, had I let her. We vied to hold him and feed him and care for him. It was hard for us to leave the baby at the end of our day shift even though we knew we were transferring him to the loving arms of the evening nurse.

After three days, the social worker came back. I carried Baby X to the waiting car and placed him in the social worker's arms. As I removed his "name tag" from his wrist and put it in my pocket, my eyes filled with tears.

Florida has enacted legislation called the Abandoned Baby Bill that provides an option for parents who do not want their newborn babies. They can leave their newborns at a hospital or fire department. There will be no questions asked. No crime will have been committed and the babies will be cared for and placed in loving homes for adoption. Hopefully, this effort has helped some Florida babies. Hopefully, it has kept some parents from leaving their infants in trash bins and lavatories or other public places to die from exposure or starvation or disease.

There is a similar law in nearly thirty-five states in the nation. I don't know how aware desperate pregnant women or couples are of the recent laws that provide a safe haven for an unwanted baby. Most expectant mothers, who know they don't want a baby but chose to deliver, go the adoption route or rely on a family member to take the child. It is the rare case, yet a reality, that you find a very scared, desperate, alone woman, often a teenage girl, who cannot cope for a variety of reasons and who abandons her baby. Sometimes it's a child having a child in a situation hard for many of us to fathom.

I often wondered what happened to Baby X. At least his birth mother or father or both had the good sense to abandon him in a safe place. The social worker told me the baby would be first placed in a foster home. After the newspaper headline, *Baby X Found on Church Doorstep*, there were numerous follow-up articles that reported dozens of families were clamoring to adopt him.

Several months after the incident my husband and I moved out of the area, and a year later my own son was born. Today, Baby X would be thirty-four. I expect he grew to be a very handsome young man. I expect his adoptive parents have long cherished him. Happy Birthday, Baby X.

CHAPTER 4

SWEET BABY BOY

BY MARY E. PELRINE

It was a sunny day in July; the kind of day a proud mother would welcome to take her new baby for a walk. But this day was beautiful in another sense. This was the day I held an angel. Marc was a sweet, blue-eyed baby who I met while working in the special care nursery. He was born in an emergency cesarean delivery at a local community hospital at 34.4 weeks of pregnancy due to a poor biophysical profile and breech presentation. Initially he was termed "healthy" with apgar scores of 9. He encountered several severe life-threatening complications requiring transfer to a specialty center. His complications included prematurity, brain damage, and heart and lung problems. He spent 10 days on a ventilator that resolved several of his life-threatening complications.

When I first met Marc, his major issues included prematurity and breathing problems that affected the composition of his blood, not enough oxygen was getting to his cells. I was eager to take care of Marc. He needed help with feeding and I spent several sessions with his mother teaching and assisting her with breastfeeding. Marc really enjoyed being close to his mother, although feeding was a struggle. He eventually learned to bottle feed, with occasional breastfeeding. He slowly weaned off tube feedings. Marc's growth was so slow that he was fed with higher-calorie milk. He was constantly monitored for breathing and heart problems. He received oxygen 24 hours a day. Several times a day, he would stop breathing and need stimulation and oxygen. These episodes worried the parents. I tried to support them as best I could. Marc recovered from his prematurity issues, but feeding, temperature instability, and growth—the issues related to his severe brain damage—persisted. The parents always visited with the hopes that their beautiful baby would not stop breathing—a signal he was improving. In fact, the episodes happened more frequently, which only supported how bad his prognosis was. It was difficult knowing this and still trying to be optimistic for the family. It was heart-wrenching to see these parents come in so sad each and every day.

Even though Marc's parents were told of, and seemingly aware of, his prognosis, I don't think it really hit home for them until we had a family meeting with our Neonatologist. I sat in on the meeting. At the meeting, the doctor was very grim; spelling out a very poor prognosis. She actually told them that she thought Marc would die. She explained how she didn't know when that would happen, but she felt his quality of life was severely compromised. Most likely, he would struggle, perhaps he would be severely handicapped. I remember so many different emotions during that meeting—feelings of denial, anger, sadness, and grief. I recall how scared the parents were—especially Marc's dad. He was frightened of taking Marc home and having him die there with no one around to help him. We all cried. I cried for Marc and the pain he might have. I cried for the parents, knowing they probably would lose their child or have a severely handicapped son. I cried for myself because there wasn't anything I could do to lessen anyone's pain.

It became apparent that there wasn't anything more our acute setting could do for Marc. The difficult decision was made to transfer him to a long-term chronic facility. Marc had a beautiful blanket that his parents always draped over him to give him a secure feeling. I asked his mother if I could take it home and embroider on it. She allowed me this honor. The next day I returned to work with Marc's name and birth date embroidered on it. Marc's mom just hugged that blanket.

I accompanied him in the ambulance to the chronic hospital. I remember telling his new nurses all about him, his history and especially what he loved most—being held. As I talked with them, I looked around and wondered how Marc would do in his new environment. He now was in a room with three other babies and a big TV. He was close to the nurse's station but there wasn't going to be a nurse in the room at all times—something I was used to at my hospital. All around me were children of all different ages, all with chronic afflictions—a constant reminder of what might happen to Marc. Marc's mom met me there and I placed Marc in his new bed. I surrounded him with "*Quakers*" (*ducks*) and his favorite stuffed animals. I covered him with his embroidered blanket and hugged his mother. I left there very sad.

When he was three months old, Marc's family made the decision to take him home. Support services were in place for them, including oxygen therapy, monitoring, and eight hours a day of nursing care. Marc's parents said that the day they took Marc home was the happiest day of their lives.

Marc's condition deteriorated and he was readmitted to the hospital. Further testing confirmed Marc's brain was shrinking. He frequently stopped breathing which further decreased the oxygen his brain was receiving. Marc's parents were faced with heartache. They took Marc home knowing at this point that they could only offer comfort and love.

One of our night staff nurses took care of Marc during the night hours so his parents could sleep. I came into work on a beautiful July day when she told me that Marc had worsened over the last day. He stopped drinking his bottle and his breathing was worse.

This particular day was my last day of work before my vacation started. I had plans after work to go shopping and buy myself a bathing suit. But I had this most compelling urge to visit Marc at home. I drove to Marc's home and rang the bell. Marc's two grandmothers let me in. They brought me to Marc's bedroom where I found his mother rocking and holding him. She was singing to him, telling him he was a sweet baby and she loved him. Marc's cousin, a cute little six-year old visited while I was there. She had waited for four months to see her new cousin and the time was finally here for her visit. She held little Marc and was so happy. I remember taking pictures of her holding him. Marc's dad was resting during this time. After this short visit, Marc's visitors left, including his grandmothers, who went to buy food for the house.

This is when I had the opportunity to hold Marc. While holding him, I could feel his breathing become more peaceful. In feeling his little chest, I could feel his heart slowing down, although it beat strongly. At this point I urged his mom to wake his dad. Marc's dad came hurriedly. I placed Marc in his dad's big strong hands. Mom and dad hugged each other as they held their son. I kept my hand on Marc's chest as I watched him take his last breath and feel that last flutter of his heart.

I watched Marc's parents as they held him close and cried for their baby and for themselves. I watched as they realized how their baby looked so peaceful, no longer feeling any pain. In the family meeting that had occurred so long ago, Dad was frightened of his son's death. Yet this day, it was dad who held Marc. It was his strength that helped Marc during his final journey. It was this moment I understood why I had this overwhelming sense to be with Marc's family on this particular day. I was there for them.

Marc was buried two days later. Several of his nurses, including me, were in attendance. Marc touched many lives during his short life, especially mine. He knew only love. There isn't a day that goes by I don't think of him.

His parents have called me an angel, but I know in my heart, the angel is Marc.

CHAPTER 5

KEELIN

By Janice M. McCoy

He was so cute; a little 5 year old boy with dark brown hair and eyes, clinging to his mom as she lifted him up into the crib. The year was 1965. I was a junior in a diploma nursing school in Iowa. His name was Keelin, and he had recently been diagnosed with juvenile onset diabetes.

I began to gather my supplies and paperwork to do his admission assessment. I had asked to take him as my case study for my pediatric rotation, which meant that I would care for him throughout his hospitalization, meet all of his needs based on his diagnosis, provide in depth teaching and instructions to him and his family, and write a lengthy case study to describe the care that I had provided during his hospital stay.

The family was poor with few resources, but they were very close. His mother Rose was very interested in learning what she needed to do to provide the best care for him when he returned home. I did all of the necessary teaching, and by the time Keelin was discharged, he was giving himself his insulin shots every morning. I taught them about proper diet and foot care, and I remember Rose telling me that she would be sure that he had clean socks everyday by washing his socks each night when he went to bed. They couldn't afford a different pair of socks every day. We developed a close relationship. I was very proud of his progress and his independence when he was finally discharged. I received an "A" on my case study and continued to progress through the nursing program.

Later in my junior year I became engaged to be married, and my picture appeared in the local paper. I received a card in the mail with a handkerchief with the words "thank you" embroidered on it. The card was from Keelin. His mom had written a note to tell me that when Keelin saw my picture in the paper, he told his mom, "That's my nurse!" and he wanted to send me a present. I still have the handkerchief that he sent me.

The first Christmas card that I received every year came from Rose, Keelin, and their family. Rose always prepared her cards over the Thanksgiving weekend and mailed them out the following week. It became a tradition for me to look for his card, and I always considered my Christmas complete when the card arrived in the mail.

Through the years Rose kept me informed of Keelin's progress. He played football during high school and graduated with his class in 1978. He worked in low paying jobs and never left the small Iowa town in which he had grown up. Several years later he married, and eventually he and his wife Barbara had three children.

Over time, the diabetes began to take its toll, and one year the Christmas letter told me that Keelin's kidneys were failing and that he was on dialysis and awaiting a transplant. He also began to have visual problems. In 1996 the letter arrived from Keelin himself to tell me that Rose had passed away earlier that year and the family was struggling to go on without her. He also enclosed pictures of his children.

Keelin's letter in 1997 broke my heart. To quote from the letter, "I found your card from last year, and it said 'Keelin, Barb, and family.' Well, it's only Keelin now. Barb left me two years ago and took the kids because she couldn't handle my disability—a below the knee amputation on my left leg. (I'm doing fine with that.) She said she wanted the kids to have a 'whole man' for a father. Oh well, life goes on. I see the kids every other weekend, and I am dating a girl from a nearby town." He also described his kids' activities and talked about what he wanted to do in the future. He signed his letter "Friends Forever." Later that year he rejected his second kidney, and had to go back on dialysis.

In 2001 my Christmas letter arrived right on schedule. Keelin was living with his high school sweetheart and their five children from their previous marriages. He told me that his son was graduating from college and one of his daughters had decided to go to nursing school after her high school graduation. The letter was happy and upbeat, and he said that he had had a "really good year."

In January 2002, less than 3 weeks later, I received a phone call informing me that Keelin had passed away at the age of 42. I was deeply saddened by the news and sent cards to both his father and his fiancé telling them how much Keelin had meant to me and how much I would miss his Christmas message of hope. My relationship with Keelin and his family spanned 36 years. I have not seen them since the day they left the hospital—a little 5 year old boy and his mom—but I feel as if he was a special part of my family and that I was still "his nurse" these many years later. I treasure the fact that we remained "friends forever."

CHAPTER 6

DINNER WITH A FIVE-YEAR-OLD

BY IDA A. SOUZA

I entered the restaurant with my husband Dale. Our son, Randy, daughter-in-law, Anne, and five-year-old grandson, Ross were already seated. I was extremely excited to see them as they had just returned from a week's vacation. Ross was coloring with some crayons and hadn't seen us enter. We went to the table. With a smile that would light up a room, Ross greeted us with hugs and kisses. Everyone seemed to be talking at once and my head was spinning. For a moment I felt overwhelmed. I sat down, took a deep breath, and tried to focus and center myself.

Ross asked several times, "Where is Auntie Kim?" Unable to sit still, he kept getting on and off the chair and turning around to check the door. The restaurant was filled to capacity. The large screen television was on. The hustle and bustle of the wait staff was evident. That's just what a five-year-old needs, lots of commotion! This certainly was a recipe for a high-tension dinner gathering. I looked at Dale and he smiled at me. A few minutes later Auntie Kim arrived. Once again, we all shared hugs and kisses. Ross asked her if she would take him to the game room. She replied with a 'yes.' We all smiled and offered her some change for the arcades.

After a few minutes they returned, their eyes alive with excitement. Ross proudly showed us the prizes he had won. He shared his trinkets with everyone. As the waitress came over to take the dinner order, Ross said he needed to go to the bathroom. Auntie Kim immediately got up and offered to take him. They returned and sat down when Ross suddenly slid off his chair onto the floor. He tried to get up quickly, banging his head on the table, he let out a howl. Anne tried to console him, but to no avail. He continued to cry while burying his head in his mother's chest. After a minute, he looked up. Our eyes met and I whispered to him, "Would you like a Therapeutic Touch Treatment?" With tears rolling down his face, he nodded his head yes.

Ross climbed down from his mother's lap still crying and looking around the restaurant. He walked over, wiping the tears from his eyes and lay down on the bench next to me. With his eyes closed, arms by his side, he looked like a little angel. Randy and Anne both gave a big sigh; the strain on their faces started to fade. Dale rubbed me on the shoulder and Kim signaled a thumbs up. I centered myself again, taking several deep breaths feeling the energy fill my lungs and body. I started the assessment and found his energy field to be imbalanced and with loose congestion. I began unruffling his entire field with both hands. As I was clearing the field, I noticed his facial expression becoming more relaxed. After clearing the field, my intentions were to direct energy for wholeness and healing. The treatment continued for approximately ten minutes. I then smoothed his entire field and grounded him.

After I did the reassessment and found the rhythm of the field had been re-established, I placed my hands on his shoulders to tell him I had finished. He opened his eyes, looked up, and asked me to do the Hand-Heart Connection. Ross lifted his little hand up to meet mine and told his parents that he knew how to do the Hand-Heart Connection. When the treatment ended, he was calm, and cheerful. He sat in his chair, like a little man, and ate his dinner and participated in the conversation. We sat for approximately one and a half hours. Ross remained tranquil and well behaved. We all enjoyed dinner and had good conversation. The outcome of this treatment was certainly a positive one. Randy said he would be willing to pay $200.00 for a Therapeutic Touch Treatment if the results were like tonight. Laughing, I said, "you don't have to mail me the check, I will take it now!"

CHAPTER 7

ALL THE KING'S HORSES AND ALL THE KING'S MEN

BY PAMELA DALEY LAFRENTZ

My year working for a Harvard Medical School neurosurgeon has come to an end. What a long journey I have taken: from the oil and gravel streets of my childhood to the hallowed halls of Brigham and Women's Hospital in Boston. What an opportunity for a nurse who, as a child, devoured library books about famous women and men of science, and actually perused the original manuscripts and case studies of Harvey Cushing, a pioneer in the field of neurological surgery.

OK—I try to avoid fits of gloom and not dwell upon the bittersweet end as there is one thing I do know: I am a nurse and opportunity abounds whether academic, research, or clinical. There is no better time to be a nurse, especially in Florida, and I will find my niche once again. Until then, I want to tell you a love story.

Susan and David waited till their late thirties to have a child. Susan quit her prestigious job at the bank, painted the spare bedroom a pale yellow, filled the room with baby accoutrements (a crib, changing table, diapers, and storybooks) and prepared for the birth of their son, Bébé.

By the infant's third day, he had totally taken over their hearts and household. The couple could hardly remember a time without him and now basked in the delightful life of parental fulfillment. And that life became a series of celebrations: his first laugh, his first back to tummy rollover, his first tooth (an event at five months that prompted a Champagne toast).

The parents devoted nearly all of their energies to caring for their baby—showering him with attention, dressing him up, and showing him off to family and friends. Bébé smiled and laughed as he played his role to perfection—

wide toothy grins for Dad as he pulled Bébé around in his red Radio Flyer wagon and loving kisses for Mom as she played *Patty Cake* and *Itsy, Bitsy Spider*.

At fifteen months Susan began to teach him the letters of the alphabet. Magnetic letters clung to their refrigerator. Large colorful foam letters lay scattered about the floor of the baby's room. Books were everywhere. While his mother read the storybooks, Bébé pointed to the pictures of moons and balloons and clocks and socks.

Her commitment was contagious; he was a quick learner. A is for Apple. B is for Bear. C is for Cookie. D is for Dada. Nearly every word they spoke to him he tried to mimic. By eighteen months he could find "middle C" on the piano. Yes, Bébé was their wonder child.

Bébé was no whiner. He usually slept through the night and eagerly consumed nearly every bite of food offered, chewing vigorously with giant new molars. Except for one isolated head cold, he was as healthy as any 21-month-old child could be. So when he became constantly fussy, many days in a row, Susan felt it was more than just teething or the approaching "terrible twos."

Pediatrician offices are often filled with runny noses or stuffy toy circus animals. Sometimes a child appears with a pea in his ear or a rash on his bottom. Susan took Bébé to her local pediatrician, remarking that the baby has been very irritable for the last several weeks. The busy pediatrician examined Bébé but could not find anything wrong with him. The doctor ordered lab work that came back normal. Two weeks later, David and Susan were back in the pediatrician's office. "Something is terribly wrong. Bébé seems to want to sleep all the time," the anxious parents declared. "He is no longer interested in taking walks or talking. And he has no appetite."

Sure enough, Bébé had lost a half of a pound instead of gaining weight like normal babies do. Once again, the pediatrician thoroughly examined him but could find no reason for concern or any focal neurological deficits. The parents had reported no seizures, although the child had vomited the day before. The infant looked normal.

The office nurse who was assisting the pediatrician looked into the suffering eyes of the two parents. Fear and frustration had replaced the animation concerning their adorable child. The young nurse, a mother herself, whispered something to the doctor. He nodded and then listened to the parents' history one more time and finally told them that he would like to get an x-ray of Bébé's head. The MRI showed a giant mass within the brain of the baby.

Within two days, Bébé was transferred to a large university hospital. He was taken first to radiology and underwent an angiogram that confirmed that the lesion was not a brain tumor but a giant aneurysm. Susan and David were stunned. They had no earthly idea that a baby could have a brain aneurysm. Brain aneurysms were for old people. A lumbar puncture detected xanthochromic spinal fluid, indicating that the giant lesion might be leaking.

Bébé was then taken to the OR, and under the capable hands of two neurosurgeons and a team of surgical nurses and scrub techs, he underwent a craniotomy and clipping of his aneurysm. Upon opening the skull, the external surface of the brain appeared normal, but the doctors noted the spider web like arachnoid was fairly stained with hemosiderin. With the help of a surgical microscope, a giant pulsating nearly 2.5-centimeter aneurysm was soon identified and completely collapsed with a titanium micro clip.

Three days post-op, Bébé was smiling, walking around his hospital room and saying, "A B C D dada mama." His mother brought him his favorite storybook, *Humpty Dumpty*. Together they read it over and over again. But his mother always ended the tale with, "All the king's horses and all the king's men, *could* put Humpty together again."

CHAPTER 8

THE LETTER

BY SUSAN GRADY BRISTOL

A letter came today. Blanketed between the bills, the vacation promotions, and credit card applications, the handwritten envelope was unfamiliar to me. The return address held no clues. I opened the letter and read, "I am the mother of one of your NICU babies from 1979." Over twenty years had past. I thought about where I was and what I was doing twenty-some years ago. A young nurse with only a year's experience, I was working in a Level III Neonatal Intensive Care Unit in the Midwest. It was the only Level III NICU within 500-miles. It was exciting work and I loved it.

Neonatal care was a relatively new field. Ventilators small enough for newborns had just been developed a few years earlier. Most babies weighing less than three pounds did not survive. Those who did were cause for great celebration. The survival of a small baby could be bittersweet. Some tiny ones ended up with cerebral palsy, blindness, or a variety of other disabilities. Yet, we continued to work with these little ones and hope for the best. One was never sure of the outcome until later. We had no official neonatal transport team, so when a call came from an outlying hospital with a sick or premature infant, we checked to see whose patients we could reassign so that a nurse could leave the nursery. The nurse leaving on the transport grabbed the tackle box filled with emergency medications, laryngoscopes, intravenous bags, tubing, and other resuscitation equipment. Someone paged the respiratory therapist who would appear lugging the small transport ventilator, oxygen tank, and tubing. The pediatric resident in the NICU came with us as we loaded up the ambulance with the transport isolette. Hopefully, the resident wasn't in his or her first year with little experience.

18

We were truly a team; relying on the knowledge and expertise of one another. Once at the referring hospital, the resident called the neonatalogist back at the NICU with a report. He explained how the baby was doing and what we had done to stabilize the baby. The neonatalogist then gave additional instructions over the phone or told us to "come on home." Before leaving the referring hospital, the nurse always stopped by the mother's room with the baby in the isolette so the mother could see her child one last time before leaving. All too often this was the last time a family saw their new baby alive.

As I read the letter today, I remembered the many transports I had taken part in all those years ago. Sometimes we rode all the way in the ambulance. If the referring hospital was over 200 miles away, we took the ambulance to the airport then hopped on a plane and flew to our destination. It wasn't until 1983 that we commissioned a helicopter for transport. By then, we were much more sophisticated and in the process of formalizing an official transport team made up exclusively of dedicated nurses.

The mother wrote that her baby boy was born in a community sixty miles away from our NICU and that I was his nurse. We must have taken the ambulance to pick him up, I thought. She had remarried, so I hadn't recognized the name on the envelope. Now I remembered the baby's name. She said he weighed 2.5 pounds at birth. She remembered some of the special things I did. I remembered the baby. He was a tiny guy, but full of spunk. On the ventilator, the tube taking oxygen to his lungs seemed to take up his entire mouth. Taping the tube in place was tricky. The tape was cut in thin strips and meticulously wrapped around the tube and secured to his upper lip and cheeks. His thin skin became raw over time from the tape. During his feisty times, he sometimes reached up and pulled his tube out. When that happened, we immediately called the pediatric resident to put it back in place. The baby grimaced and tried to cry around his tube whenever he was upset. I comforted him with a little music box or by stroking his back or chest. He seemed to recognize my voice as I opened the portholes of the isolette and bent down to talk to him.

Since his mom and dad were unable to visit very often, I wrote letters from the baby every few weeks and "signed" them with his footprints. Bath time was my favorite time with the little guy. Even with all the tubes and monitors, I managed to take him out of the isolette briefly and hold him while another nurse changed his bedding. If he was stable enough, I sat in a chair and rocked him and talked to him. The NICU nurses did that with all the babies. This baby was just as special as the rest. My 2.5-pound patient stayed in our unit for a little over two months. He grew stronger each day, weaned from the ventilator, started oral feedings, and was moved to a crib. I don't remember his dismissal specifically. Over the years, there were several dismissals. The parents were always excited, a little nervous, and anxious to get on with their lives as a family.

In her letter, the mother thanked me and proceeded to tell me how her adult son was now 6 feet tall and is finishing his Master's Degree at the university. She included pictures of him as a baby, as a little boy around age 10, and as a high school graduate. "Thank you for the care you gave him 24 years ago," she wrote. "I just wanted you to know that this baby grew up to be a wonderful young man."

CHAPTER 9

THE UNSMILING VISITOR

BY KIM CECCARELLI

Kathy, the case worker from Children's Services, knocked on my clinic door one morning. I had just arrived to start my day as the school nurse for an elementary school located in one of the poorest, most crime-ridden neighborhoods in Dayton, Ohio. Kathy asked if I would be present while she talked to one of the students she had been working with over the last six months.

"Of course, Kathy. Who is the student?" I inquired.

"Her name is Sarah Hazard and she is a sixth grader here. Do you know her?" Kathy asked. "No," I answered. As the school nurse, I was responsible for the well being of over 600 students. I didn't know all of them personally.

Kathy quietly filled me in on Sarah's family history of sexual abuse by her father. Mr. Hazzard had also sexually abused two older twin sisters who presently were living far from the nightmarish home, both pursuing college educations in California. None of the girls would openly implicate their father in the abuse, so he was still living in the home with 12-year-old Sarah.

Kathy's explanation was interrupted when Sarah knocked on the door. Sarah was invited to sit down and chat. Kathy greeted her warmly and introduced me as the school nurse. Sarah was a somber looking African American girl with pigtails and large soulful eyes. There was no preteen silliness that other girls her age typically exhibit. When Kathy asked her questions regarding how things were at home with her father, Sarah lowered her head and said softly, "Things are fine at home."

One of the first things I learned about Sarah from that visit and subsequent visits to the clinic was Sarah volunteered very little about herself and her family. She was serious—much too serious for one so young. She never smiled. The meeting between Sarah and Kathy was over in several minutes and not much progress had been made in helping Sarah escape her abusive home. Without her cooperation and disclosure to law enforcement officials, Children's Services was unable to help her. I am sure Sarah still loved her father in the confusing and incomprehensible way children always love their parents, even abusing ones.

The following week, Sarah showed up at my clinic door. "Hi Sarah. How can I help you today?" I greeted her with a big smile. She came in silently, sat on the cot, and took off her shoe. She uncovered a painful burn on the top of her right foot, about three inches wide and four inches long.

"Sarah, how did you get that burn?" I asked her gently.

"I was making coffee for my daddy this morning before school and I spilled it on my foot," she said with little emotion. This incident glared at me as another example of the "wife" role this child was assuming at home. In a perfect world, the father would be cooking Sarah's breakfast before she went to school. I cleaned and dressed Sara's wound and asked her to return the next day so I could check her burn.

After she left for class, I called her father to verify Sarah's story. Mr. Hazzard stated that Sarah was clumsy that morning while she was getting his coffee. I asked him if he would please take her to see a physician to assess the wound further. He refused saying, "She'll be all right. She don't need no doctor."

I saw Sarah everyday to redress her burn and to check on the healing process. I instructed her on simple first aid. I asked her to refrain from walking barefoot or getting the burn area dirty while playing outside. I taught her how important it was to keep the burn clean and to use safety when cooking at home.

During these many sessions with Sarah, I gained a little of her trust. She would never talk about the specifics of the abuse she endured at home, but she let me into a little bit of her world. She told me of her older twin sisters who wanted her to join them in California. She told me about a relative who bought her ticket to California to visit her sisters. Then she told me about her plans to visit her sisters in California over spring break. Sarah was planning on not coming back.

Spring break was a week away. Her father had agreed to allow Sarah to visit her sisters in California. I spent time with her everyday, inspecting and caring for her wound. The wound was healing slowly. I told Sarah she would have a scar on her foot. I taught her how to clean and dress her wound so she could take care of herself. I gave her some first aid equipment and some stamped envelopes with my address so she could write to me from California. I gave her some money to buy food on her trip. Finally I gave her a cross to wear around her neck. I asked her to write to me and gave her a big hug as she left my clinic. I prayed God would keep her safe.

Spring break ended and Sarah never returned to school. I prayed fervently that she was okay. I was kept very busy tending to the needs of other students. Finally, one day a letter arrived at my house. It read:

Dear Nurse Kim,
I arrived in California... I like it here. Please don't tell my dad where I am.
Love,
Sarah.

I never saw or heard from Sarah again. I can only hope that she is living a happier life.

CHAPTER 10

MARTIN MAKES THE TEAM

BY JUDITH DORWARD

I first met Martin when he was in third grade. Martin was not like the other children in the neighborhood. His skin was white in a neighborhood where most boys had brown skin. He was taller than the other boys and awkward. On the playground most of the boys spoke a language he couldn't understand. At home his older sister, Katrina, who was much more outgoing, dominated the shy Martin. She made fun of him whenever she had the chance. Martin had a secret, though, that made the hard parts of his life a little softer. He was in love with his third grade teacher.

Martin's mother had a difficult time as a single parent. Eventually Martin was put into a foster home. When he was in high school he went to live with his father who had remarried and had several smaller children. Martin adored his little half-sister Becky. The family moved frequently and Martin changed schools often. Sometimes they were homeless.

When Martin enrolled in the high school where I was working, I was thrilled to see that he had managed to stay in school, though it was hard for him. He was often tired from working to help support his family. He didn't quite fit into this school either. Never athletically inclined, Martin had put on weight. He had no hope of making the football or basketball team. He didn't have the time. He had to work. Martin had a bad case of "teen-aged skin," at a school where one pimple meant a trip to the dermatologist for most students.

Martin had another secret. He created a family for himself at school. Mr. North, the auto shop teacher, was the father. Martin took as many shop courses as he could. He visited Mr. North before and after school. I became his school mother. Martin knew which days I came to his school and was always ready to help carry my equipment in from my car. He liked to tell me things Becky had said or ask for advice about little things. One day he dropped into my office to tell me about his plans for after graduation. Martin was going to be a Marine. He took all the tests and passed.

He came to school to say good-bye before he caught the bus. He was a scared, overweight, awkward, pimply boy getting on that bus. He had never had a date or a girlfriend—had never really belonged anywhere.

Several months later I looked up from my desk. There was Martin—home from basic training! He had come to school straight from the bus stop to see his shop teacher, his counselor, and me. He was a totally different person. Here was a handsome, fit young man with a clear complexion and confident posture. He loved the Marines. The discipline, the challenges, and the hope for a future had left their mark on Martin. Every girl in the hall turned to look at the handsome young Marine in his new uniform. Martin had found his team!

Chapter 11

BRIAN

By Kathy Hageseth

One 3 o'clock to 11 o'clock shift, I cared for Brian, an 18 year old with a severe head and neck trauma, who was in the very restless stage of his head injury. His mom, a nurse, was with him. She stayed much of the time and did a lot for him. She and I bonded immediately, not only as a nurse and the family of a patient, but also as two moms. In the couple of weeks following the accident, Brian had not followed commands or spoken. He had just been transferred back to our intensive care unit from rehabilitation after respiratory distress from inhaling the tube feeding formula. He even needed to be placed on a ventilator overnight, and was not breathing on his own. Brian's mom felt he was really focusing on her and he had begun to occasionally say 'yes' and 'no.' He continued being restless, however, to the point of almost perpetual motion, broken only by short naps that only energized him for the next few hours. When you have taken care of many head injured patients, you have a feel for the patient's real personality, even in the light of restless kicking and thrashing. There are naughty kickers and restless kickers. Brian was definitely in the latter category, the kind of kid who would never hurt you on purpose.

Brian's mom needed breaks, so as often as I could, I offered them to her. She was gone, and I was sitting by Brian's bed, holding his hand and dodging thrown beanie babies and flailing legs. He was looking right at me.

I said, "What is your name?" Slowly and hoarsely, he said, "My name is Brian."

With a lump in my throat, I asked where he was. He said, "In the hospital." I just couldn't wait until his mom got back. When I told her, we both teared up, and I said that it was a birthday of sorts for him. Brian mumbled something, and his mom asked, "Brian, when is your birthday?" Without much pause, he looked at her and said, "February 17th." Brian had a long way to go, but he was back—and I give thanks for being privileged to stand once again on that holy ground that surrounds our patients and their families.

Chapter 12

Bottoms Up

By Janice M. McCoy

Jeannie was 16 years old. I was 19 and a junior in nursing school when I was assigned to take care of her following a serious car accident. She had been riding with friends and was thrown from the car when they lost control on a country road. She landed face down in a ditch, and the car's muffler and tail pipe came to rest across her buttocks. She was unable to move away from the hot metal, which proceeded to burn almost 3 inches deep into her entire backside from hip to hip.

The year was 1965. It was summer in the Midwest, and the weather was glorious. Unfortunately, Jeannie's injuries would require an extended stay in the hospital and painful treatments to prevent infections and promote healing. My assignment as a student nurse was to care for her and to gain skills and competencies in the treatment of burns, care of an adolescent, and all of the challenges that a teenager has to deal with during that time of her life. The medical ramifications of a burn, including electrolyte imbalance, immobility, and potential scarring and disfigurement were real possibilities.

I was somewhat overwhelmed, certainly scared of what I would be required to do, and challenged to care for someone almost the same age as me.

Burn treatments in the 1960s consisted of silver nitrate dressings, zinc oxide ointment, skin grafting, and isolation. Silver nitrate is a clear liquid that was delivered to Jeannie's room in clear, plastic, liter bottles. It looked like water, smelled like water, and was the consistency of water.

It turned everything it came in contact with black, however, and all of the table surfaces and floor tiles were spotted with black stains wherever the liquid had spilled or dripped during the dressing changes. Zinc oxide is a white paste that was applied to the burns with wooden sticks that looked like overgrown tongue depressors. All of Jeannie's care had to be delivered while garbed in a sterile gown, mask, and gloves to prevent any exposure to contamination and possible infection. It was hot, tiring, and painful for both of us, but a bond developed between us, which gave me great confidence in my journey to becoming a 'real' nurse.

Jeannie was forced to lie on her stomach with a sheet suspended over her bottom by a metal cradle which prevented the bed linens from laying on her wounds and causing pressure and discomfort. We had to rig up a table-like apparatus to allow her to read, eat her meals, and play games or other distractions to pass the time. Her school provided a tutor for her so that she wouldn't fall behind her classmates in her schoolwork. Using a bedpan was agonizing for her, and we were also challenged to find a way to pad the bedpan without soiling her bed and causing embarrassment and possibly contaminating her wounds. There were constant challenges while encouraging her independence, keeping her occupied, and at the same time protecting her from additional harm or injury.

Jeannie was very popular and had a lot of friends who came to visit and sent cards to wish her well. Her boyfriend was a constant visitor, and we taught him how to put on a gown, mask, and gloves so that he could enter the room and spend time with her. Her wounds slowly healed over a period of several weeks. My rotation ended, and I moved on to another unit. Jeannie was discharged to resume her life, a bit older and a lot wiser for her experience.

Moving ahead to the summer of 1973, I was now an RN and had worked in Labor & Delivery for approximately five years. My husband had been laid off from his job, and we had returned to our hometown where I was working nights at the hospital where I completed my training while he searched for a new job.

One night while I was on duty, a patient arrived on the unit in early labor. I escorted her to the admission room and proceeded to start her admission process. I timed some contractions, asked the initial admission questions, and gave her a patient gown so I could move her to a labor room and make her comfortable. As I was assisting her to remove her clothes, she turned her back to me, and I immediately noticed a very unusual sight—she had a deep, curved burn scar across her buttocks. My first words to her were, "I know you!" I was embarrassed to think that I had recognized her by her bottom and not her name! It was Jeannie! We were both so excited to see each other, and I was also glad to see her husband who had been her boyfriend at the time of her accident. They had married and were there for the delivery of their first child. What a privilege and an honor it was for me, as a nurse, to once again play a pivotal role in the life of this family.

CHAPTER 13

MARIA

BY PATRICE E. HARRIS

Years ago, a young girl, Maria, was admitted to Mercy Hospital following a car accident. She had severe head trauma. A neurological assessment showed she did not react to pain, her pupils were dilated and fixed, and she was draining grey matter from her brain. She was not expected to survive. Her family refused to take her off life support. She was finally moved from the intensive care unit to a special care unit. I did not expect to see her again. I thought she would gradually deteriorate and pass away.

Several years later, I was placing my order in a Burger King when a young woman asked if I was Pat. I said yes, and she said she was Maria. I nearly fainted. I couldn't think of what to say. She invited me to come to see her baby. I sat down and gathered my wits. She said she remembered me because I kept her going the first few weeks after the accident. She said I never shut up. I talked to her all the time I was taking care of her. She said I always told her what I was going to do before I did it. I told her what her family was doing and thinking, and what day it was. She even remembered me shaving her legs and underarms.

I always thought a patient can hear when in a coma, so you must talk to them. I did it out of habit with Maria, not completely sure she could hear me. I learned an important lesson and I hope that all nurses will give all of their patients hope by talking to them—no matter their condition.

CHAPTER 14

NO ORDINARY JOE

BY AMY S. COGHILL

How can I even begin to describe my experience as a nurse with Joe? I do know that, in the end, I was able to stand back and reflect on my role in his cancer experience and on my growth as a nurse over the last three years. In retrospect, I feel that my role in his care did not fit a traditional description of nursing responsibilities, but rather transcended those boundaries. It involved the interactions and connections of the soul, the care of the physical body as a system, and the concern for the frustrations of the mind in the face of severe illness.

He was thin, articulate, and radiant (by 'radiant' I mean he exuded a positive light, rising from the soul, palpable when you entered the room). Joe needed a bone marrow transplant for acute myelogenous leukemia (AML) at the ripe age of 18. He graduated high school and went to his prom all in the same day before he came to us. I quickly signed up to be his primary nurse, not just because of his beautiful qualities, but because he said I was "nice." He mentioned several times that he felt comfortable with me as his nurse. I even got applause from him on occasion and eventually went on to hold the title of "favorite nurse." I felt that with this trusting relationship I could do a lot of good for him.

Joe came from a family of six other brothers and sisters. His independence, insight beyond his years, and love for his family were dramatically apparent in his interactions with me. I knew these were resources I should respect and could also use as positive reassurances should he need to look to them for strength. I connected with Joe better when I sat down and just talked eye-to-eye, friend-to-friend. He wanted straightforward information about his progress and where things were headed. He made this very clear to me one day when his frustrations were high. He vented exactly how he felt about the situation he was in, his discontent with his doctors, and how he felt he was being inadequately treated. Concerned, I sat and listened to his feelings pour out. His requests were simple and simple to remedy. I took some time to reassure him that I would provide him every morning with his white blood cell count (WBC) so he could track the engraftment of his new stem cells. I offered simple yet thorough explanations of all bedside procedures and stayed at the bedside with him for comfort during them all (first femoral catheter placement for renal dialysis, abdominal ultrasound). Because Joe's mother had to take care of all the other children during the daytime hours, Joe was often without any family at the bedside for support during these anxiety-producing moments. My presence offered Joe reassurance and assisted him in learning about his current physical situation. He was not afraid to ask me questions and felt better spiritually and mentally when he was more informed.

No matter how horrible his mucositis (severe destruction of the lining of the GI tract from chemotherapy, including the mouth, which often develops several days after the last dose of chemotherapy) became or how jaundiced he got each day, he always said he was doing fine. One day I walked into his room and found him drooling uncontrollably into his emesis basin, strung out on a Dilaudid PCA (which I subsequently decreased due to his increased somnolence and confusion). Despite his obvious discomfort, he refused to focus on his pain, instead saying, "Oh, hey! Are you my nurse today? Good." I'd ask him how he was feeling—if he was hurting—and he genuinely answered, "I'm fine. My mouth's bothering me, but otherwise, I'm great." And he meant it! As our nurse/patient bond grew, Joe just kept on shining. Such an enduring, positive soul was Joe's most valuable resource.

I don't think he knew exactly how infectious his spirit was. Joe inspired me as I went about my physical nursing responsibilities for him including staying on top of his fluid status, lab values (I was responsible for repleting his electrolytes per standing orders based upon the low values I found), need for numerous blood products (required to decrease anemia and assist in coagulation), infection control (the BMT population is profoundly neutropenic and at great risk for infection), central line dressing changes, pain control, need for rest, diarrhea management, and nutritional status. I made time to teach Joe and his Mom about what to expect when he got home, how to take care of himself once discharged, and the need for daily clinic visits. These multifaceted physical aspects of his stay with us and his endurance with this disease were overwhelming at times, but, at the end of the day, he'd reassure me that he felt things were going well.

As the transplant course went on, Joe required large amounts of platelets, fresh frozen plasma (FFP), and cryoprecipitate infusions. Though patients who require bone marrow transplant require multiple infusions of blood products, I knew his liver could be failing due to the need for such frequent amounts of FFP and cryoprecipitate. Joe was at a significant risk for uncontrolled bleeding.

I watched his creatinine, bilirubin, and blood pressure climb daily. This concerned me as I knew that increased creatinine levels could indicate kidney dysfunction, and that increased bilirubin might indicate venous occlusive disease (VOD) or even graft versus host disease of the liver (the phenomenon of the newly implanted bone marrow/stem cells of attacking and destroying the host organs, namely the gut, liver, and skin). Prognosis for reversing these system failures in the bone marrow population is ultimately quite poor, especially in someone as young as Joe.

Despite me sharing frequent bad news, I also had the pleasure of talking and laughing with Joe and his mother, listening to their life story together. Joe even let me read a short story he wrote for his school literary magazine. He was very proud of his work, as it won a prize from the teachers and was placed right in the middle of the magazine. Family was Joe's favorite subject. He knew his siblings very well and spoke of them often. He had their personalities, likes, and dislikes down to an exact science. It was Joe's dream to become an elementary school teacher. He enjoyed teaching his two younger sisters and told me they missed him while he was in the hospital.

I walked into his room one morning after being off for a few days and I saw this amber-colored kid saying, "Oh yeah! You know today is going to be a great day. I got some sleep last night, my throat is a 4/10 (pain scale rating), and I feel good." All of this he said in a kind of "Yippee!" tone. I had to chuckle and again was stunned that, in the face of such a bad physical picture, he felt fine, even improved, and rejuvenated. I felt horrible because I had to lay the news on him that we had to get an ultrasound of his liver to see what could be wrong with it, and a chest x-ray to make sure he wasn't bleeding into his lungs. We also had to get some more FFP and platelets dumped into him, and then we had to be ready to have a femoral line placed for his first dialysis. I felt like the ultimate squelcher of all that was positive in Joe's morning. I even sensed that now his positive energy could be a cover for his extreme fear. I made an extra effort to stay at the bedside with Joe all day. I arranged a change in the assignment with the resource nurse who quickly reassigned my other patient to an accepting colleague.

The day was hectic beyond belief. Joe got weaker and quieter. His mother had arrived at the bedside that afternoon. Then, twenty minutes before he was to complete his first dialysis treatment, he said to his mother sheepishly, "I'm scared." For three weeks everything had been okay because Joe said it was and willed it so. He scribbled, 'I love you' on a Post-it note. He wanted all of his siblings and family to read it and to know it. I felt like he knew something I didn't know at that moment. I knew the picture was bad from the physical data and presentation, but the acknowledgement of the spirit and mind hit home hard. I left his room for a moment and went into the lunchroom to cry.

The next day I got a call at home on my day off saying Joe just got transferred to the ICU. I came immediately that evening to see him and his family. I spent two hours talking with his mother and their priest before we went back to his room, where we talked for another hour at Joe's bedside. We each held one of Joe's hands and watched him lie there intubated and quiet. His mom showed me the last words he scribbled on a Post-it note earlier that day before the transfer. It said, "All is well." And again, for me, it was.

Joe died about one week later surrounded by a cocoon of love and family in the ICU after an unyielding battle. About ten of Joe's family members stood around his ICU bed holding hands and praying at the moment of passing. At that precious, quiet moment, I stood there holding the hand of Joe's brother, who donated the stem cells, and the hand of Joe's spiritless body. I felt like the symbolic bridge between the two brothers.

Joe's spirit continues to live beyond his illness and rubbed off on all of us involved in his life. I can't describe what a privilege it was to be a part of it all. Even in the face of death, I knew that if he could talk to us, he would've said, "Hey guys, it's okay! Don't cry! I'm going to be all right. And I love you." I couldn't help but feel a glow inside even at the moment of passing. I knew "all was well."

Though I've been officially a nurse for only a short time, I have learned (from what seems to be several years of complicated situations) countless lessons. These situations and lessons have made me more than just a Clinician III, but a better person. So, what's the moral of the story? In other words, what have I learned, not only from Joe, but also from all of the other patients I've encountered during the past three and a half years? It's not about how many IVs you can start successfully or how well you can dress a wound. It's not about being detached from your surroundings and peers and practicing in a vacuum with nice, neat, little protocols. It's more about whose life you touch and who touches yours. It's about daring to feel all emotions when you truly care for your patients. It's about listening to people, even when you can't understand the "whys." It's about going forward from the beginning to the end of a patient relationship, despite the rocky course. It's about wanting to care for people because it's a good thing. And above all, it's about sharing yourself, not just at work, but wholly and genuinely throughout your life.

CHAPTER 15

WHAT A DAY

BY VIOLET HORST

It was a Monday morning and I had just returned to work following a three-week vacation. My assignment consisted of caring for four young patients. The first was in kidney failure and was on overnight peritoneal dialysis. The second was a three-month-old, hospitalized with chronic diarrhea due to in-flammation of his colon resulting from premature birth. He was receiving in-travenous nutrition as well as tube feedings into his stomach. The third patient was hospitalized with infectious viral bronchitis and was on contact-isolation precautions. The fourth patient was a 17-year-old with cerebral palsy and mental retardation who had a sitter with him because he was so restless that he could hurt himself. In the daily patient report, the charge nurse mentioned the need for caution when approaching this last client, due to his pinching and hair-pulling behavior if one got too close to him.

After the daily patient report, I briefly checked the charts to get a clearer picture of my clients and of their recent health history. When I entered the room of the client on dialysis, the mother began a lengthy interrogation about my knowledge of kidney failure and the use of dialysis. The disease questions were easy to answer but since it had been a few years since I had worked with dialysis, and this was an updated model, I had to appear more confident than what I felt. However, Mom eventually heaved a sigh of relief, seemingly satis-fied that I had passed her test.

As I entered the room of the infant with diarrhea, the two-and-a-half-year old in the other bed announced, "He smells yucky." My patient's explosive diarrhea had overfilled his diaper, contaminating most of the surrounding surfaces. By the time I finished cleaning the baby and his surroundings, an hour of my shift had elapsed. I had not even glanced at the other two clients. Rushing into isolation, I overlooked my own number-one rule in approaching toddlers: allow them time to accept my presence. As a result of my hurried-ness, the toddler yelled "Get away from me, I hate you!" Offering soothing words, I did a rapid assessment and continued with a flow of comforting phrases as I exited the isolation room.

Assuming that the sitter of my fourth client would have alerted me if that child had an unusual need, I had left him until last. As I entered the room, the sitter urgently asked me for relief for a quick break. Recognizing patient-care assistants have elimination needs, I immediately granted the request and turned my attention to the client. Indeed the shift report had been accurate: this severely-handicapped 17-year-old was quite restless. As he jumped out of bed and darted toward the window, I attempted to keep the IV pole mobile and synchronized with his movements. After he flung himself back into bed I brainstormed about how I might calm this very frightened individual. Singing came to mind, and although my repertoire only consisted of a few lullabies, it proved successful. As the client calmed down, I became braver, sat on the bed and lightly touched him. However, when I stopped singing he impulsively grabbed and pulled my hair. Wanting to be free of pain, but not wanting to use undue force, I reverted to problem-solving mode. Again I sang but this time I added clapping in hopes that he would mimic me. Much to my relief he let go of my hair and clapped.

I wish that I could say that things flowed smoothly for the remainder of the clinical day, but that was not the case. Each hour brought new opportunities for problem solving. This is what makes nursing challenging, satisfying, and never boring.

CHAPTER 16

A GOOD HAIR DAY

BY JUDITH DORWARD

It's Friday! Almost the weekend, and I have a plan to catch up. I'm far behind in my work, but if I don't allow any distraction, and work really hard all day, I can do it.

The door to my office is closed and I hear kitten-like mewling from behind it. "It's Tabitha," the secretaries inform me. "The significant other has been beating up on Mom, and Tabitha's upset. She wants to go home. We put her in there so she can't escape."

I open the door. Nine year old Tabitha is not an attractive child, especially with a really red, swollen, and blotchy face. Her hair is uncombed, stringy, and matted. Her hands really need scrubbing, but she managed this morning to find jeans and a sweater that aren't too dirty.

"I hear you're having a bad day, Tabitha," I acknowledge.

"I want to go home! I want my Mommy!" she wails.

I let her cry for a little while before I offered, "Bad days happen, Tabitha, but sometimes they aren't quite so bad if you have good hair." I rummaged through my stash of combs, barrettes, and hair ribbons. "I don't think braids are quite the thing," I said, combing out her snarls. "Maybe high pony tails." The crying subsided as we worked on her hair. By the time we were finished, the sniveling had stopped. "Have you had breakfast?"

"No, I didn't want to eat. I want my Mommy."

The secretary ordered breakfast for Tabitha from the cafeteria. A donut and chocolate milk and applesauce. Not exactly health food.

"You know, Tabitha," I said to the munching child. "Bad things happen, and sometimes we can't make those bad things go away. But sometimes we can try to make special things happen, and then the bad days aren't quite so bad."

As if on cue, Brandyce appeared in my office announcing, "I'm here to have my head checked." Brandyce had been sent home for head lice.

"You know, Tabitha, I think Brandyce might need special hair, too. What do you think?" We agreed that an asymmetrical ponytail might be just the 'do.' Out came the combs, barrettes, and hair ribbons.

Head check and hairdo completed, Brandyce invited, "Let's go play, Tabitha." There were ten minutes left before class. They headed out the door, hand in hand, each armed with a new comb in their hip pocket.

"You have the same ribbons. You must be twins," I said. I hoped that Tabitha would always remember the power of good hair and a good friend for turning a bad day into something special.

CHAPTER 17

WHO DOO-DOOED THE WORM?

BY JUDITH DORWARD

Is there a job in the public schools less understood and less appreciated than that of custodian? Custodians are sent to clean up every yucky mess that children can produce. A suspicious noise somewhere? The custodian will take care of it. A small boy in need of male guidance? The custodian will take care of that too.

Friday, 1:30 PM. School is out in an hour. Nancy, the yard duty lady, storms into the office. "There's a worm in the girl's bathroom," she announces. "Send for Ed. I'm not touching it!"

The secretary rolls her eyes. "Come on Nancy, a little worm. How hard can it be?"

"It's a big worm and I'm not touching it! It's not in my job description!"

The secretary sends for Ed, the custodian. He appears with heavy black rubber gloves. I might as well go along, I think. Something in this cries for the attention of a school nurse. I think of my physiology professor, a parasitic helminthes nut. Surely his student could not pass up the very slim chance of an exotic find. I empty the Band-Aids out my jar and tag along. Never send one public employee when you can send three.

We enter the girls' bathroom. Sure enough, draped across a toilet seat is a ten-inch long worm. It looks a lot like an earthworm, but it's much bigger and paler, and is pointy on each end.

"Looks like a human intestinal parasite to me," I announce as Ed gingerly scoops the worm into my Band-Aid jar. I slam the top down on the lid and wrap the jar in paper towels. No use starting panic on the playground. I feel like Beverly Crusher with an alien life form.

There are 500 kids in the school. School is out in less than an hour now. I need to find out exactly what this worm is, and exactly which of the 500 doo-dooed it.

I drive very carefully to the Health Department Lab. Getting stopped for a ticket would eat into my precious time. Health Department employees are fascinated. "Maybe someone is playing a trick," offers a lab tech. A public health nurses announces, "It's a round worm! I had a patient cough up one just like it in the emergency room. You need to find out where it came from. That kid needs treatment."

They relieve me of the worm and promise to call me once they have an exact identification. "I want my jar back," I say. "Just disinfect it first."

Back to school. Five hundred kids. I can't very well threaten to lock down the school until someone tells who doo-dooed the worm. They'd never tell. We have to use logic. It has to be a girl; so we are down to 250 suspects. "It has to be a fourth, fifth, or sixth grader," offers the secretary. "They were on the playground then." That leaves 100 suspects and less than 20 minutes.

Desperately, I grab the class list book. "Let's try girls who have been in refugee camps." Only six. I speak to the girls, one at a time. We discuss the importance of telling the truth, even if it might embarrass you, or you think it might get you in trouble. Or you think somebody might get mad at you. The first girl, Pang, knows what I'm talking about. Oh, yes, I heard about the worm, but I didn't do that kind of potty. It wasn't me," she assures me. The other five girls haven't the faintest idea of what I'm talking about. We have our suspect. I send En, Pang's older cousin to talk to her. Less than five minutes left.

En returns just as the bell rings. She confides to me, "Pang says that a worm was trying to go up her butt. She is real scared. She won't tell anyone."

Friday afternoon. 2:40 PM. School is out for the weekend. The worm has been identified. Pang and her family will be treated.

Ed is disinfecting the girls' bathroom.

CHAPTER 18

THE HARDEST JOB I HAVE EVER LOVED

BY AMY BARNES

It is 7:00 am and I am entering my "Thursday" school and getting myself mentally prepared for the day. As a school nurse with an assignment of four schools (two elementary, one middle, and one high school with a combined population of over 5,000 students), it does take some time to get "reprogrammed" for each new day. This is one of my elementary schools and as I walk into the office, I see the normal morning hustle and bustle. I enter the clinic and pick up my folder where my invaluable clinic assistant has placed my mail, updates regarding student concerns, the weekly report, and other miscellaneous papers. I hear taps on the window as students begin to stream by and wave on their way to class. The clinic door opens and the day begins!

In rolls one of my most medically fragile students. He is a wheelchair-bound fourth-grader who has a tracheotomy, continuous oxygen, and an infectious smile. He wants to tell me all about his recent fishing trip sponsored by the "Make a Wish Foundation." It is great to see him so animated and full of excitement. He, of course, wants the weekly update on how my dog, Lucy, is and he tells me that he will draw another picture of her when he comes back later in the morning for his treatment. Other students begin to arrive with medication refills, notes from parents, and clinic passes. My clinic assistant brings us both coffee and we attempt to catch up on a weeks' worth of information as we tend to the children's needs.

Ah, the life of a school nurse; kissing boo-boos and putting on Band-Aids. Ha! Not quite! I am always amazed when I talk to parents, teachers, and other individuals in the community about how little they understand the role of the school nurse. I describe it as one of the hardest positions I have ever loved.

Today's school population includes an increasing number of children with significant health problems; some of them life threatening. The nurse must be someone who can function well as an independent practitioner. Interpersonal skills and the ability to be an effective communicator are a must since the nurse is working with children, parents, medical professionals, faculty, and school administrators. The nurse must also have exceptional assessment and problem solving skills since we do not have the availability of sophisticated medical technology at our immediate disposal. Flexibility and organizational skills are critical and I have also learned to trust my gut feelings.

Who would have thought that as a school nurse I would be involved with more emergency life-saving interventions than I was in all my years as a hospital-based nurse. I have often said that one day I would write a book entitled, "I Couldn't Make This Stuff Up If I Tried!" I could never have predicted that at the very beginning of one school year, I would be faced with a seventh-grader who came into the clinic complaining of a stomachache. It turned out that this young lady had recently had a baby and her C-section incision was opening up because she was lifting weights during her Physical Education class! Just the fact that she had recently had a baby and was recovering from a surgical intervention was a shock, not to mention that none of this information was communicated to the clinic. Or how about the student who for some inexplicable reason decided to cut the ear lobe off of another student during class. Let me tell you, the ear really bleeds! Not only are we there for the students, but one time an individual from the neighborhood came running into the school office with blood all over her. She had reached into her closet and severely cut her arm on a broken piece of glass from a picture frame. I have no idea why she came to the school but it just so happened that I was there. I held pressure on her wound with a sanitary pad, the most absorbent item I had at my disposal, until she was able to get the medical attention she needed. Trust me, the list goes on and on. Not only are there the physical issues to address but the emotional and psychosocial needs are incredible. I remember telling my husband that at times I feel like I am in the Peace Corps in my own community.

As I take a sip of coffee, the clinic phone rings. The person on the other end of the phone identifies herself as an employee of the Epidemiology Department of the Lee County Health Department. The individual goes on to say that a student at the high school assigned to me had died in the early morning hours from the disease, Bacterial Meningitis. She asked that I go to the high school and find out which students may have been in close contact with the deceased student and might require prophylactic antibiotic therapy. I felt my stomach twisting but instinctively my mind started with the questions; had "Student X" been to the clinic the previous day and if so, what were her complaints? Who were the student's teachers and how many classmates may have had close contact and require treatment? What did I even remember about Bacterial Meningitis? And, of course, I thought about how tragic this was for the student's family. ALL I KNEW WAS THAT I HAD 17 MILES TO PUT A PLAN TOGETHER!

I quickly got my things together and told my clinic assistant that I was needed at my "Friday" school and to page me if anything came up. I threw my "office in a bag," (suitcase with wheels), into the trunk of my car and grabbed my resource books from the backseat to quickly refresh myself on the disease. Thank heaven for cell phones and the fact that I kept a phone list of all my schools in the car.

I called my "Friday" school and asked to speak to the principal. I shared with him the news that I had received from the Lee County Health Department and that I needed to get the names of the close friends of "Student X." The principal indicated that he would email only those teachers who taught the deceased student and he would carefully word it so as not to cause any alarm. The names were to be sent to my email address. I also asked the principal to advise the guidance counselors of the situation at hand and to please locate an office where I could meet quietly with individual students. I assured the principal that I was on my way to the school and that I would come to his office as soon as I arrived to further discuss our plan of action. I also contacted my clinic assistant in the high school to let her know that I was coming there and that I would update her when I arrived. I then phoned my supervisor to advise her of the situation and what steps were in place up to that point. She immediately assured me that she was on her way to help with this enormous and emotionally charged task.

It was now 8:20 am I arrived at the high school and quickly went to see the principal. His secretary provided me a copy of the email that had been sent. The guidance counselors soon arrived. I summarized the information that I had gleaned from my medical resources as well as the information provided to me from the Health Department. The biggest concern from the counselors was how the disease was spread. I reinforced that since the disease is transmitted through droplets from the secretions of an infected person, unless an individual had had a recent "saliva exchange" (kissing, sharing food, drinks, lipstick, cigarettes, etc.), the likelihood of transmission was very small. I then shared my immediate priorities which included, identifying those students who may have had close contact with their deceased classmate, interviewing those individuals to determine their level of exposure, and informing the parents as to their child's "risk status" and treatment recommendations. This information then needed to be communicated to the Epidemiology Department so that they would know how many doses of medication would be required. The Health Department was also putting together informational letters about the disease, which would be sent home that afternoon with each student. They were also going to send an individual to assist with a faculty meeting scheduled for after school. In addition, arrangements needed to be made for the availability of grief counselors as well as a central information center because once word got out, there would be a barrage of questions from students, parents, faculty, and the press.

It was now shortly after 9:00 am and my supervisor arrived. She went to speak with the principal and the other administrators and I headed to the clinic. When I shared the circumstances of this tragic situation with my assistant she was devastated. She told me that "Student X" had not been in the clinic at all that week. I shared with my assistant that I would be giving her the names of certain students whom I would need for her to call down to the office that I was provided. I also told her that she would need to be prepared for a busy day because once news got out, there would be many students coming to the clinic for comfort, information, or both. I checked my email and the teachers had sent me the names of 17 students. I pulled their emergency cards so I would have phone numbers to contact parents and I grabbed a few boxes of Kleenex. My supervisor and I then headed to our quiet space where we discussed our strategy in meeting with each student. We agreed that we needed to be compassionate, but at the same time we needed to get specific information quickly and determine whether or not there was a real risk of a recent exposure to the disease. Once we gathered the information needed, we would then contact the student's parent to advise them of the situation and provide the parent with an opportunity to ask us questions. Since we had many students to meet with, once we obtained what we needed and provided information and comfort to the student, they would then be taken to a guidance counselor for additional emotional support. We took a deep breath and felt that we were ready to call for the first student.

Each session was difficult. We calmly explained that their friend had become very ill the previous evening and had passed away in the early morning hours of Bacterial Meningitis. We explained how the disease was transmitted and asked if they had shared any food, drinks, lipstick, cigarettes, and so forth with their friend within the last few days. As mentioned earlier, we needed to ascertain this information quickly before each student reacted emotionally. We then called each student's parent to give them our opinion as to whether or not their child was a candidate for prophylactic antibiotic therapy. Parents were encouraged to contact their personal physician. Most parents came to the school to comfort their child and to get reassurance from us. Upon completion of our first round of interviews, it was determined that seven students would require medication.

During the time that we were meeting individually with the original list of students, the principal made a general announcement, to the school staff, that a member of the student body had passed away that morning from Bacterial Meningitis. Students who had a concern as to whether or not they may have been exposed to the disease were instructed to report to the clinic. Students were also encouraged to see their guidance counselor if they required any kind of emotional support as a result of hearing this very sad news. Kids poured into the clinic and the front office in a range of emotional states. Again, my wonderful clinic assistant was able to provide some order to the chaos and additional grief counselors were available to assist in the clinic.

The day was an emotional blur. Had it not been for the coordinated teamwork and support from the school and community resources, I am not sure how we would have made it. Informational notices about Bacterial Meningitis were delivered to the school as well as the required medication permission slips. The Health Department informed my clinic assistant that she was to collect the signed permission slips the following morning and then the medication, which was to be delivered by the Health Department, could then be administered. Parents were given the option of receiving the medication from their personal physician if they preferred.

The school day was over and it was now time for the mandatory faculty meeting. Again, information about how the disease is spread was shared and staff were reassured that their risk of exposure was extremely low. Many questions from the staff and faculty were asked and answered by the experts from the Health Department.

What a day! All of us involved spent some time after the faculty meeting together to debrief. We discussed what worked and what did not. Our major recommendation was that for future crises, it would be better to communicate to teachers via email what the circumstances were. This would allow each teacher to share the knowledge in a more personal way with their students. Teachers would be notified via an announcement to check their emails. I offered to put together a protocol based on our recommendations should such a situation ever occur again. This protocol is now part of a school nurse manual used by all school nurses in our state.

As I reflect on the events of this day, I am overwhelmed. I am convinced that what I learned from the Nursing Process as well as my nursing experience, gave me the structure I needed to make it through. My skills in assessing, critical thinking, planning, decision-making, communicating, implementing, and evaluating were all put to the test. As a school nurse I have learned that there is no such thing as a typical day. It is challenging, frustrating, and rewarding all wrapped up together. It is the hardest job I have ever loved!

CHAPTER 19

IN THE SCHOOL NURSE'S OWN WORDS

By Anne St. Germaine

Often enough I hear school district administrators talk as though the major task of the school nurse is to provide first aid and Band-Aids. I usually try to help them to understand that first aid, which can be taught in less than a week, has to do with stabilizing life when a person has a life-threatening accident or event. I also try to tell them that the major task of the school nurse is triage. It takes years to learn which "sick kids" need a nap, which need a listening ear, which ones need a doctor's appointment, and which need a trip to the emergency room.

Then, the decision of how to follow up is not simple either. Do they need a Band-Aid or referral to a specialist? Who calls the parents? Should the nurse contact the doctor directly?

Since most education administrators stop listening half-way through my explanations, I have searched for a way to hold interest while they have a chance to fully understand the complexity of the nurse's task. The following true accounts from school nurses in the Seattle Public Schools demonstrate the breadth of their practice.

Chris Mochel, Elementary School Nurse

When he transferred into the Seattle School District as a third-grader, Anthony's mom said that her son used to be allergic to peanuts when he was little. She said, "He probably isn't allergic anymore because he can eat one peanut occasionally and it doesn't seem to hurt him." I told her about allergy tests and insisted that it was important to his safety for her to get accurate information about his sensitivity to peanuts. Over winter vacation she did take him to see an allergist, and on the simple screening test he tested for a negative reaction. This mom told the clinic what I had said about a more accurate test and demanded it be done. They returned to the doctor the next day for this testing and Anthony did show a dramatic response to peanuts. The doctor recommended continued caution about ingesting any peanut products. Thoughtful patient teaching helped this mom to become a strong advocate for her high-risk child.

Maureen Rigert, Elementary School Nurse

One of our third grade students brought gifts of necklaces back from Mexico and gave them to six of her friends at school. Most of the necklaces had mercury inside a blown glass chili pepper pendant, which hung on a black cord. One morning I noticed one of the necklaces was slightly damaged and the mercury was leaking out in small amounts and getting on the hands of three girls. We later learned that several students had significant amounts of mercury stuck to the soles of their shoes. By the time I found out what was happening, the classroom and the library were contaminated with mercury. I called the Seattle Poison Center and the custodian called the school district hazardous-materials coordinator. The Poison Control Center informed us that such a small amount of mercury was not alarming. They suggested that each child wash the areas of skin that touched the mercury. The hazardous-material coordinator arrived within an hour. We also invited the PTA president, a marine biologist with a machine that can detect mercury in fish, and scanned all the kids we identified as possibly contaminated. In the end, we confiscated three pairs of athletic shoes and one shirt, which was disposed of by the hazardous-materials coordinator. I then sent a group e-mail to my school nurse colleagues, recommending that they be on the lookout for these necklaces. They are illegal to sell in the US, but travelers may bring them home as souvenirs or gifts. Teachers aren't trained to recognize these potentially poisonous "gifts" and we were all relieved to learn that the danger could be minimized with simple interventions.

Patricia Salazar, Kindergarten through 8th Grade School Nurse

Recently, a second grade teacher approached me about a student who kept "spacing out" several times a day in class. David was not responding and seemed to be staring into space. When questioned, his first grade teacher verified this behavior although he could not remember how often or how long this had happened. I called David's mother stating that I thought he might have absence seizures and that a visit to a neurologist would be in order. She was very reluctant, saying, "There is nothing wrong with my son. He just "loses it" once in a while. And I don't know any of those doctors anyway." I told her I was worried about David falling behind in class, because he would miss important information that was being taught. She agreed to take him to her regular doctor. This was a start. As it happened, her regular doctor referred David to a neurologist who observed that, during an EEG, David had three seizures. He is presently on medication. His seizures are decreasing as his medication reaches a therapeutic level. Absence seizures are easy to miss and we were lucky to catch this one early for David's sake.

Liz Terry, Elementary School Nurse

I have an 11-year-old student, Al, who can be a handful! He always seems to be looking for routes of escape from the classroom. Al and I have a good relationship, so he often visits the health office. Al came in one morning complaining that he did not feel well; he was coughing. He was not coughing in my office; in fact, he was chatty. It would have been easy to dismiss his complaints. I asked a few questions about his coughing. "Do you cough at night? Does coughing at night disrupt your sleep?" He didn't feel feverish, but he had a temp of 101 degrees. When I listened to his lungs I could tell that there was no air exchange in the middle and lower lung fields. He said he didn't feel tired at all! This was an episode of as yet undiagnosed asthma. He had never had an asthmatic episode before then. We caught it before it could affect his attendance and learning.

Shirley Swindler, Middle School Nurse

Mike is a sixth grade student who is quite bright and very articulate. He has problems with Attention Deficit Hyperactivity Disorder and also with Anxiety Disorder. He has received medication at school intermittently depending on his individual therapist's orders, but is on medication from home daily. Mike's teachers and parents (one parent is a teacher) have agreed that Mike can come to the nurse's office as a respite if he needs a quiet spot to regain control. The nurse is someone he is familiar with (due to medication administration) and Mike experiences the nurse's office as a quiet and safe spot. There are times when Mike needs a quiet time with no talking and times when he needs to discuss options and alternatives. One day, Mike was distressed and came down for a quiet time with the nurse. He also interacted with a health assistant assigned to the school that day. She sensed that Mike was upset but did not feel comfortable dealing with the situation. Her interactions were appropriate with Mike but she deferred to me to help Mike. I was on the phone and unavailable and Mike left the office. The situation was heightened when he came back between periods later in the day and handed the health assistant a letter he had written. She looked at the note just briefly and handed it to me, as it was a poem expressing suicidal ideation. I retrieved Mike from the classroom, called his mother and sat listening to him, talking with him, and watching him cover his head and curl up and cry at times. When Mike's mom came, she was upset, needing some emotional support and comfort in a private area. You can't call a nurse to come in for this situation from somewhere else. The student and mother both needed help and they needed it on the spot. If a nurse was not available, or there was only a health assistant (as many would propose for budget reasons), how lost that person would be in this situation.

Mary Stone, Elementary School Nurse

I became a school nurse so my work schedule would closely match that of my children. What I found was the assessment and communication skills required for the job are very challenging. The health assessments and neuro-logical assessment were much more comprehensive than what I did admitting people to the hospital.

The school nurse is the only health care practitioner in this setting and often there are significant findings. The school nurse is the only one in a position to find these problems. Referring children to other medical or dental services is a daily occurrence, but sometimes the problems we find can be very serious. Preparing staff to respond to emergencies and anticipating po-tential problems for individual students require nursing skills I had not used before. I feel like a detective, trying to discover the details of those students with serious health concerns.

Recently, I completed a physical, neurological, and vision assessment for a child who suffers from Post Traumatic Stress Disorder. Talking to the mother was a challenge because she did not want to discuss the painful details of what had happened. After obtaining her trust and providing emotional support, she was able to share the details of her son's experience; not only the critical incident, but other events, which shaped his reactions to his teachers. I was able to help the teachers to understand this student better. I was also able to help the psychologist with her diagnosis of his learning disability.

First aid and Band-Aids are a very small part of my job. The teachers and secretaries frequently provide Band-Aids, even when I am present in the schools. I have had many challenging jobs in many years of nursing, but being a school nurse has been the most challenging one for me so far. I have to stay current on many health-related topics. I find the work very fulfilling because I can see that I make a difference in the lives of students. I don't have enough time at each school to do all that I know needs to be done for the students' health, but I do what I can with the time I have.

Connie Craig, High School Nurse

Bob is a twelfth-grader who suffered his first psychotic break this summer and spent most of the summer in hospital inpatient care. He has trouble taking his medications and is in foster care. I have spent many hours with this student and in conferences with his doctors, nurses, therapists, teachers, and vice principal. Bob required a specific care plan as well as a disability accom-modation. This required interfacing with his mental health worker as well as his foster parent. In November he began to show signs of a relapse into schiz-ophrenic behavior. He was delusional, confused, not sleeping or eating, and acting in a bizarre manner both in school and at his foster home. He was refusing to see his mental health worker or take his medications. I contacted the mental health professionals in an attempt to have him hospitalized. They refused to hospitalize him, as they did not feel he met the requirement of a danger to self or others. I worked with Bob within the system for another month until I was able to have him agree to be voluntarily admitted to a well regarded inpatient mental health unit. When he wanted to leave the hospital, I consulted with the emergency room psychiatric resident. Later, I appeared in court to support his involuntary treatment procedure. Since that time he has been released and will be coming back to school for our second semester. He will require continued skilled nursing support to maintain himself safely in the school setting. However caring they may be, educational staff have neither the time nor the expertise to diagnose psychotic behavior and support a student through his making a voluntary commitment for hospitalized mental health services. Nurses can assist by providing this critical liaison.

Barbara Hopp, Elementary School Nurse

Mary is a diabetic third-grader. She had been recently diagnosed. It took a while to teach her to manage her diabetes within a narrow range of blood sugar. I don't believe that a teacher or a nursing assistant could be expected to make the subtle and important decisions about how to treat a young, newly diagnosed child. I needed to call her parents about either a very high or very low blood sugar X times in October, eight times in November, and six times in December. Three of these times she needed to take insulin. The brain is the body organ most sensitive to the level of sugar in the blood. There is no way that Mary can be learning in the classroom during times when her blood sugar is in such poor control. She needs a practiced eye on her condition as she learns to manage it herself. It is my role as the school nurse to monitor Mary's condition to make sure she is unimpeded by her diabetes in the classroom.

Mara Lankow, Elementary School Nurse

I do a lot of teaching with elementary school students who have chronic health conditions. Tanya, a fourth grade student, experienced crisis-level symptoms of asthma last spring and was hospitalized in the intensive care unit for several days. The family is Somalian and as recent refugees into this country, language is a barrier. I was informed about Tanya's diagnosis and kept teaching and re-teaching her about her medications and performing and interpreting the meter that measures her oxygen intake. Throughout the spring months I was in contact with the home health nurse and the doctor on a weekly basis, and faxed the oxygen readings to the doctor monthly. With the start of school this year, I have made home visits to Tanya and am continuing support and treatment. I have referred her to the doctor for emergency visits twice this year. On her own, she wasn't letting her mother know when she was having trouble breathing. I know that the relationship we have developed has been very helpful to her and has prevented many hospitalizations. Being here three days a week has also been critically important. Seeing her once a week would not be enough to help her interpret the changing patterns of her oxygen meter readings and breathing levels.

Maureen Rigert, Elementary School Nurse

Students who have recently entered the United States begin school at a Bilingual Orientation Center (BOC) in our school district. The school nurse is often the first source of health care these students have had in a long while. Health screening frequently reveals the need for medical or dental follow-up, and the nurse routinely gives families information about Medicaid for children at the same time as referral to community health settings. One such student failed the hearing screening portion of the assessment. The nurse sent a letter to his family, along with Medicaid enrollment information in his language. The family applied and was approved. The boy subsequently was found to have severe damage to his middle ear and complications following years of un-treated middle ear infections. He had surgery and now wears hearing aids. It is easy to imagine that adapting to his new country would have been much more difficult if we had not made this discovery early.

* * * * * * * * * * *

As you can see from these stories, nurses in the schools are not optional. Ask any of the parents whose children's lives were changed because of something the nurse alone noticed. Ask any principal or teacher who has had to call 911, unsure of whether a situation was life-threatening or not. I am proud to be associated with the nurses who tell these stories.

CHAPTER 20

SLEEPING THROUGH THE NIGHT

BY JEAN SHEERIN COFFEY

Why do some patients touch your heart and stay in your mind? I wish I knew. After 26 years of nursing I can say with assurance I have interacted with hundreds of children and their families. Each child touched my heart in their own special way. Each child had a name, a story, and made an imprint on my life. So why do some make a bigger imprint than others? Why do some stay in my mind for years? I do not know the answer but I want to tell you about one young lady who left an everlasting imprint in my heart.

Tonight I was watching the news. It was a usual night, cleaning the supper dishes and half listening to the local news team tell me the day's events in the Champlain Valley. I was loading the dishwasher and glancing at the screen. I saw a familiar face of a young lady who has crossed my path many times in the past 17 years. There she was on the big screen getting a nebulizer treatment and chest physical therapy. She is all grown up. Why is she on TV? Quick, turn up the volume—I need to hear her story. All I heard was "rushed to the children's hospital . . . . Her family said she is doing better."

Oh no! Melissa—what is going on? I need to know. Is she OK? I run to my address book and dial up the hospital two states away. I am put on hold. The minutes go by agonizingly slow. Memories begin to flood my mind.

It is January 1987 and I am just getting to work for the night shift on the pediatric unit. Driving to the hospital in a snow squall, I thought about my three children (ages 4, 6, and 7). I had tucked them in to bed before I left for work.

When I worked nights I arrived hoping many of the little kids were settled for bed as best they could be. As I made rounds, chest tubes, IVs, and dressing changes illuminated the sharp contrast between the kids I left at home and the ones with whom I would spend the next eight hours. Melissa was one of those kids not quite ready for sleep. She was newly diagnosed with Cystic Fibrosis and this was her first admission to the pediatric unit. She was part of a heavy assignment this shift and I wondered how the night would go.

I found her very awake and asking lots of questions. Her mom was very attentive but had that exhausted look that comes with days and nights of vigilance at the bedside of a sick child. Mom was apprehensive. She was far from home and maybe overwhelmed with so much to learn about this complex disease. Both mom and Melissa were wary of me, the new nurse. I introduced myself to mom and Melissa and I played with her toys for a few minutes.

Mom was learning how to care for a child newly diagnosed with CF: medications, chest physical therapy, and intravenous medications. How overwhelming this must feel. A lifetime of care ahead and it all started a few days ago. I strongly encouraged mom to take a night off and sleep through this night's medication administration. Daytime was a fine time to learn and she really needed to get some rest. Mom was reluctant at first. I could tell she was not sure if she could trust this new nurse to do the job.

I helped mom get settled on a cot by the bedside and tucked Melissa in for the night. Sleep came fast for the two of them and I continued my work for the night. Melissa needed intravenous antibiotics at the same times. It was a busy night and the early morning brought an emergency life threatening event that resulted, in this case, in death.

Mom and Melissa slept all night and awoke refreshed and surprised I had not made enough noise to wake them. I cared for them several more days before they headed home to life in farm country. I often thought of them.

That spring, the hospital magazine arrived in the mail. I was getting ready for work and quickly scanned the articles. Pediatrics was featured this quarter. I saw articles about many of my esteemed colleagues. I turned the page and there was a picture of Melissa's mom. A *Mother's Diary* was the title that graced the top of the page. I began to read the journal entries. The entry for January 15 began with "Jean Coffey was our nurse tonight and she is just super. I never even heard her at 4:00 am."

I was touched. I had been a nurse 11 years and had not felt this proud. I also felt incredibly humbled. This journal entry changed my life. I realized that I was touching lives. Despite the long hours and challenges of being a pediatric nurse I made a difference for kids and families. During the course of my career I have often gone back to that diary entry when I questioned myself or needed to be reminded how blessed I was to be a pediatric nurse.

Over the years, many children with Cystic Fibrosis made frequent appearances at the pediatric unit. Melissa did not come often but when she was admitted I tried to provide her care. I learned about her passion for cows. She became an expert at showing beef cattle at the county fairs. Her name appeared often in the local paper and I followed her progress with great interest.

Several years passed and I changed my job. Sadly, I lost touch with Melissa. Years later I returned to the pediatric inpatient unit as the director of the Children's Hospital. It was during this time that Melissa and I got reacquainted. I heard about the cows, basketball, and saw how she was growing in to a beautiful young lady.

In 1996 I was asked who I would nominate as the Children's Miracle Network (CMN) Champion for the telethon that year. The telethon is a yearly event to help raise money for children's hospitals nationwide. The telethon champion becomes the spokesperson for the local children's hospital. Melissa immediately came to mind. She was now an articulate young woman who often advocated for children with chronic illness. The CMN telethon committee agreed with the choice and I was able to be the one to tell Melissa and her mom about the honor.

The excitement that followed her appointment included a trip to Washington DC to meet Socks the cat and President Clinton (in that order of importance according to Melissa). A trip to Disney to meet Donnie and Marie Osmond followed. A TV appearance on a national station was included. She was caught up in a whirlwind of activity and took her role seriously. She did a phenomenal job.

That spring, Melissa co-hosted the telethon with me. We had so much fun interviewing patients and talking to the guests. One of the hockey players from the local university, Eric Perrin (now a NHL star), surprised her by arriving at the show. He had become acquainted with her during one of her stays on the pediatric unit. She was presented with a hockey stick on the air. It was an electrifying moment during the broadcast.

For one whole year she and I spent time at fundraising events. I got to hear about her aspirations for college. I also heard her disease was beginning to change her life. She was not playing basketball now. The cows were harder to show and she was not sure she could go away from home for college, but she would try. Her first choice was Northeastern University in Boston. That was my alma mater.

The next fall I was in Boston when I heard she was accepted to Northeastern. I quickly ran to the bookstore and purchased a window sticker for her car. I put the sticker and a long letter in the mail. I was in Boston and she was in farm country—our lives parted again.

During the next few years I left Boston and Melissa went off to college. I often wondered how she was doing. I never got around to writing like I wanted to do so many times. During those years one of my own children became ill and had open heart surgery. Best intentions to keep in touch crumbled under life's daily pressures.

Now, as I am on hold, I am asking for one more chance to hear her voice and talk to her and her mom. I am so afraid of what I will hear back from the nurse on the other end of the phone. As a nurse, I often took these types of calls, frantic friends and family members anxious to check on a loved one.

The words I hear are music to my ears. Melissa had a lung transplant and she is on the step down unit, doing well. The nurse sends the call to Melissa's room.

Mom answers the phone and we chat like we just had coffee together last week. I get all the details about the last few years. Melissa never finished her first year at college; she got too sick. She moved home and her health continued to deteriorate. She had lost so much weight; she was a mere 80 pounds before surgery.

Now the good news: today she is doing well. Chest tubes are coming out, her spirits are good and she is hopeful for the future. Just as I started to say "tell her I say hi and give her a hug . . . ." Mom says: "OK here come the goose bumps—Melissa wants to talk to you."

Yes the goose bumps arrive and at this moment I know why I am a nurse. On the other side of the phone I hear that sweet voice, "Hi," she says. 'Hi' spoken with new lungs. We talk for a minute.

Twenty-six years of nursing, gallons of tears over children who left us, boxes of Kleenex, hours of laughs from children who looked illness in the eye and spit at it, sleepless nights wondering what else I should or could have done, millions of pages read to try to make me the best pediatric nurse in the world. The hours at the bedside with joy, fear, pain, laughter, awe, and exhaustion. Tonight I feel I now know true fulfillment in life. Goosebumps and all, I have been blessed with a gift from a girl who slept all night so many years ago. I know I will sleep all night tonight.

Thanks Melissa. You have taught me about spirit, perseverance, love of family and friends, and, most of all, that we should cherish every day and live life to the fullest. I tell your story to countless pediatric nursing students every year. Your legacy will live on and I thank you for the gifts you gave me.

Post script: Despite a valiant fight with Cystic Fibrosis, Melissa died on June 1, 2004. You will be missed, Missy!

CHAPTER 21

THE YOUNG MAN'S FEET

BY HAZEL MARIE BARMORE WIEGERT

In November 1998, I was working at the Augsburg Central Nursing Center, located in the basement of a local Lutheran Church. The Center was open Sunday and Monday mornings, and Tuesday afternoons. The Center was staffed by registered nurses employed by Augsburg College, students, and volunteers. I was participating at the Nursing Center as part of a graduate nursing class. At the time, the staff gave away many socks and personal toiletries.

One morning, a young man came requesting some foot products and a pair of socks. I asked if I could look at his feet. He told me that he had not changed his shoes or socks for three days. I was not sure what to expect. He was homeless, 27 years old, and had had wet feet for three days. He said that he thought I should wear gloves when I touched his feet. I was down on my knees looking at his feet. I have never seen feet like his. The skin was very white and looked like it could slough off. The odor was very foul, making me nauseous. I was unsure what to do. I asked him if he would like to soak his feet and have a foot message. He thought that would feel good.

I prepared the soak with some disinfectant and oil. After he soaked his feet, I massaged his feet with some lotion and gave him a new pair of clean, dry socks. At the Center, we had a voucher system with a local drugstore for patients to get some over-the-counter items. I wrote the voucher for some special foot items. He said he could go to a friend's home to soak his feet. I told him he needed to get his feet healthier so that he wouldn't get an infection. He understood that he was too young to have bad feet. Living on the street required sound feet. He had been an athlete in high school and understood his needs. I told him the hours that the Nursing Center was open and urged him to return so we could check his progress.

He returned to the Center the following Monday. I checked his feet and they had improved 100%. I had him soak his feet and gave him a massage. He told me his friend said with feet like his, he should just cut them off. An elderly male volunteer asked me if I had seen the young man's feet. I said I had seen them and they were much improved over last week. The volunteer thought the feet still looked awful. I gave the young man another pair of socks. He thanked us and called us angels. He left the Center that morning on the road to recovery, I hope. He has not returned again.

CHAPTER 22

INFORMED CHOICE

By Page M. Vandewater

"You hate me!" Elaine glared at me from her bed as I came through her door to listen to her bedtime prayers. "You're mean to me," she raged on. "You make me wear *this*," as she pulled the tube bringing her oxygen out of her nose. "You're mean and you hate me!" The verbal assault knifed my heart and froze me in place. Elaine, an utterly delightful person with Down Syndrome had always treated me with love and kisses. She was usually willing and able to negotiate life's bumps and bruises.

My immediate response was emotional. Mentally, I angrily told her in no uncertain terms, "You have no choice, Miss Elaine. You must wear oxygen 24 hours a day!" I managed to bite my tongue before these words slipped out of my mouth. I knew an angry explanation from me would be like throwing gasoline on burning embers—turning a small fire into a conflagration.

Elaine, despite her disease, had survived to the nearly unheard of age of 67 years. She also had a congenital heart defect that never had been corrected. At this point in Elaine's life, oxygen was a requirement. It was a necessity if she was to remain alive. Elaine enjoyed her life. Although mostly homebound, she lived in a loving home where she spent her days doing puzzles, calling the family Bingo games, entertaining her company, and enjoying her favorite TV shows. She could walk independently and did her own care. My perspective was that wearing oxygen 24 hours a day, seven days a week was a relatively small price to pay.

But it is not my body and not my choice to make.

I had to resist the temptation to say, "I do know best. Do what I tell you." It was critical that I find a way to let Elaine understand the "risk-benefit" issues:

the annoyance of the oxygen versus death. As I pondered how to do this in a respectful way and in a way she would readily comprehend, my eye fell on a framed picture of her and her beloved brother-in-law, Si.

A-ha! Inspiration immediately struck me like a bolt of lightning. Si had recently died and Elaine wept copiously over her loss. In accordance with Jewish tradition, Elaine lit a candle for 24 hours and placed it next to this picture. Additionally, she had kissed the picture of Si repeatedly lamenting the good times they would never again share. Elaine had also placed flowers on Si's grave, braving temperatures too cold for her health and dragging the oxygen with her. She also traveled to a family member's home to sit Shiva one night.

I saw I could use Si's death as a "word-picture" to illustrate to Elaine her choices. "Elaine, sweetheart," I said as I sat down on the edge of her bed. "I don't hate you. I love you with all my heart. I am not making you wear this oxygen. You can take it off if you want to, and never wear it again."

Elaine stared at me round-eyed in utter disbelief. She couldn't believe her ears. Other times when she had mildly complained about the oxygen, people had always made a funny remark to redirect her, and she would put the oxygen tube back into her nose. This was the first time anyone had told her it was okay to remove it.

I stroked her cheeks as I gently said to her, "No one *makes* you wear this oxygen. You wear it because you *choose* to. If you don't want to wear it you can leave it out and that is okay."

Elaine continued to stare at me incredulously.

"I want to explain to you what will happen if you do not wear your oxygen," I continued. First you will feel a little weak. (Before she had oxygen, she did have a seizure when her oxygen level in the brain got very low.) Next, I will call the ambulance and you will go to the hospital. Then you will become weaker and weaker. Finally, you will die. The big black car from the funeral home with all the flowers will come to the hospital to get your body." I had Elaine's undivided attention as I spoke. "Then all of your relatives and friends will come to the funeral home. They will look at you in the casket and cry. Everyone will sing hymns and say prayers. Then the men will carry your body in the casket outside to the big black car with flowers." I still had Elaine's undivided attention. "We will go the cemetery. When we get to Si's grave, we will stop. Next to Si's grave the men will dig another big hole. Then the men will take the box and your body and . . . "

"Stop! Stop! Elaine sat bolt upright and pressed her soft hand over my mouth to stop my story. "That's enough. Never mind. Give me the oxygen." Elaine put the tubing back in her nose and never complained about oxygen again.

The important thing was Elaine did have a choice, as do we all. What meant so much to me was that I was able to phrase the "risk-benefit" issues in a format that Elaine could understand. She, like everyone else does, was able to make her own choice based upon accurate information.

CHAPTER 23

FINDING HOPE

BY CATHERINE THOMPSON

The medical floor on which I work is primarily for patients with HIV. I usually see patients in the last year or two of their life, as their white blood cell count drops—often into single digits—making their body susceptible to many diseases that a healthy body is able to fight daily. During these years, patients are often discharged and readmitted, becoming commonly known among the nurses as "frequent fliers." We know their story, we know their families, we know how they contracted the disease, and we know who in the family still does not know they have HIV. We are happy to see the patients we like the best, but we are upset to see them readmitted—the more often they come in, the closer we know they are to death.

People outside of my hospital continue to surprise me with their ignorance regarding HIV. When I tell them I work with AIDS patients, many are shocked. Sometimes, I can see fear—even in nurses' faces—which I find upsetting. I remind them that in many ways I am safer than most people because I never presume anyone, no matter how healthy they look, doesn't have HIV. Nurses who work with few or no AIDS patients sometimes become casual and forgetful about taking necessary precautions. I can never afford to be careless.

Miguel is one of my favorite "frequent fliers." I haven't seen him in a few months. His face lights up when I walk in the room. "How 'ya doin' baby?" he asks in a tone I never find condescending, just sincere.

"I can't complain. How are you doing?" I ask. I visually scan to see the outline of a skeleton under the sheets. He looks thinner than his last admission, if that is possible. He suffers from chronic diarrhea, which is very common in HIV patients. His hemoglobin and hematocrit are plummeting again, and the doctors fear he is bleeding internally. I will have to give him multiple transfusions tonight and place a large IV catheter in his bony arms—I cringe at the thought. "You're getting too skinny," I try to tease. "Are you eating?"

"I can't, honey. As soon as I eat, the diarrhea starts," he says. His eyes suggest frustration. Food is often a solace to many, but in his case, it has become a menace. I don't know what to say. I ask Miguel how things are at home, and he tells me that the social worker wants to put him in a nursing home, but he doesn't want to go. He lives by himself. He will need an increase in homecare services, and I hope Medicaid will pay for it. His legs are too frail, and he is unable to ambulate farther than the chair pulled right next to his bed.

"Tonight is going to be a good night," I promise him. "Once you start receiving the blood and some fluids, you will start to get some of your strength back." It's the only short-term hope I can give him. I often tell patients and families that we will take it one day at a time. When death hovers so close, the future can become unbearably frightening.

"I'm just so happy you're my nurse tonight," he grins.

I walk out of the room feeling a tightness in my throat, which I swallow hard. I know that soon, Miguel won't be discharged from the hospital. He will be one of the many patients I see die in their forties and early fifties. HIV robs countless people of their elder years. Parents bury their own children. Many of the people I care for were IV drug abusers. They were addicted to the life of the street, and if they die as active users often their "friends" desert them. They are buried in an unmarked grave. Many times, the patient's significant other is also HIV positive, and is afraid of his or her own future. As a nurse, I believe I have an obligation to provide hope and to discuss unresolved issues—before it is too late.

In the morning, before I go home, I find Miguel's doctor beginning her day. I remind her that he will need to see a nutritionist, a physical therapist, and possibly a psychiatrist to prescribe an antidepressant. The doctor is concerned about whether or not he received his blood transfusion, and what his most recent vital signs are. I tell her that he received his transfusion without any complications, and his vital signs are stable. I have done my job for the night. The patient is physically stable, but I know Miguel's spirit is slowly decaying. His hope is fading.

I walk back to the room to wish him a good day. He is sleeping soundly, and I walk out of the room, feeling my own exhaustion from being up the whole night. Curled in the fetal position, his spine protrudes from his thin skin. He looks like the pictures I see of Holocaust survivors, or people starving in developing countries.

Strangely, I feel peaceful. The morning light is a reminder of a new day—one I would normally take for granted if it weren't for my patients that remind me that a new day should never be taken for granted.

CHAPTER 24

A GENTLEMAN WHO TOUCHED ME

BY LYNN COLETTA SIMKO

Mr. Obert was a 60-year-old gentleman who I grew very attached to over the two twelve-hour shifts that I worked with him. He was a large gentleman, about 220 lbs and six feet tall. He was admitted on a Friday night via a helicopter transport to a coronary care unit near Pittsburgh, PA with heart failure and a possible heart attack. The heart attack was ruled out but he was indeed in heart failure. He was also not putting out any urine, which is not a good sign when a person is in heart failure.

About three weeks prior to his admission, he experienced a bug bite of some kind to his right elbow which became infected. He was admitted to a local hospital in Ohio for an incision to drain the infected elbow. Further testing showed a staph infection. He was placed on intravenous antibiotics. With additional technology, he could go home and continue the antibiotics. He planned to move in with his loving daughter who would oversee the antibiotic administration. But before he could be discharged, he developed the heart failure, and was transferred to us for further treatment.

This was the first hospital admission for this otherwise healthy man. He was very devastated that he had fluid building up in his lungs and was finding it difficult to breathe. He was fitted with an oxygen face mask. Although the mask made it difficult for him to communicate, he began to tell me about his life. He had two children, one son and one daughter, and five grandchildren. His wife died approximately two years ago. She was ill with cancer. He delivered all the care she needed, including bathing her, toileting her, medicating her, and most important, loving her. It appeared that he had suffered a great loss with his wife's death. But then he went on to discuss his grandchildren who he doted over. He told how one grandson would call him first thing in the morning to place his order for pancakes for breakfast. Mr. Obert and his grandson had breakfast together every school day waiting for the school bus to come. He spoke lovingly about his children. The children demonstrated their love by staying in the waiting rooms until Mr. Obert was discharged. They were very impressed with how he cared for their mother and never left her side. The children wanted him to know he was not alone and that he could count on them.

As it turned out his heart failure was caused by kidney disease. When the kidney stops working, fluid accumulates in the body and in the lungs. This kidney disease was caused by his bug bite and the infection that ensued. Mr. Obert was very sick and weak. He was receiving multiple intravenous medications to control his high blood pressure and to help increase his urinary output. Additionally, there was the possibility that he would need to be put on a ventilator to help him breathe.

The second day I was caring for him was the worst day. He told me that he would be with his wife soon. This comment took me off guard. I sat down and talked to him at length about what he meant by that. He said that he had never been sick in his entire life. He did not even have the energy to sit up in bed, let alone eat anything. He felt that he was dying. I couldn't let this gentleman think that he was going to die soon. I explained that this condition is usually short-lived. With the proper antibiotics, we would get his infection under control. We could use dialysis to clean his blood of the waste products. With his blood "clean," his appetite would return. I told him it was not time for him to see his wife. I thought, 'she is looking down at him right now and praying he will get the strength to fight on. After all, who was going to make breakfast for his grandson when school started in four weeks?' He then asked me if I could arrange for him to see a priest. I called Father Hoffman who was on call for the hospital, and told him about Mr. Obert. He said he would come in. Father Hoffman talked to Mr. Obert for about 30 minutes, gave him the sacrament of the sick, and communion. Then he went to the waiting room and talked to the children, who were very grateful to him.

I did not see Mr. Obert for five days because I was not scheduled to work. I called in to see how he was doing every other day. When I returned to work he had been transferred out of the coronary care unit. I went up to see him in his new room. He was sitting next to the window in a recliner chair with no oxygen mask. His face lit up when he saw me. He said, "You know you were right, I am starting to feel better." I found out that he was no longer receiving dialysis and that they were planning to discharge him in the morning. He still needed intravenous antibiotics so he was still going to move in with his daughter temporarily. His son was in the room; his daughter had run to the café for something to eat for lunch. They had not left his side the entire hospitalization. Tears came to my eyes as I said good bye to Mr. Obert and his son. They had touched a very special place in my heart. As I left, Mr. Obert thanked me for the talk that we had in the coronary care unit.

CHAPTER 25

SOMETHING TO SMILE ABOUT

BY STEPHANIE F. CHOMOS

Some years ago, and I won't say how many, I was working in a rural community hospital in northwestern Pennsylvania. I had been out of nursing school for about six months and was in charge of the night shift. There were a Licensed Practical Nurse with medication privileges, a nurse's aid, and myself caring for 20 patients on a normal night.

Hospital policy stated that rounds were to be made every hour on the night shift. The licensed staff usually shared this task. Early in the shift I came across an elderly male patient trying to climb out of bed and seeming very anxious. I entered his room and asked what I could do to help him get more comfortable and rest.

With a tremble in his voice he said, "Why, I've lost my dentures!" It was early October and getting cold at night in that part of the country, so he was wrapped in a number of blankets. By this time, they had been stirred enough to look more like a pile with this little gray head sticking out the top. I began pulling away a few of the blankets and was worried the dentures may fall and break on the hard floor. I told him to try to get some rest, and I would be in before leaving in the morning to help him look some more. He was comfortable with that, and was restful on my next few sets of rounds.

At about 4:00 am as I was passing by his room, the gentleman was up in bed with the lights on. When he saw me entering he waved frantically and said, "Say, I found my teeth!" "That's wonderful!" I said. "Where were they?" His reply? "Why, they was bitin' me in my butt!"

I completed my night giggling and he slept.

CHAPTER 26

BEING A NURSE

BY GRAYCE MASSI-VENTURA

It's 6:30 in the morning and the benchmarkers are here again today. They are efficiency experts that are helping the hospital improve effectiveness and time utilization in the preoperative holding area and the operating room. I have my three patients. I'm the Clinical Educator. I'm extremely well organized, and I'll have no problem getting my patients admitted and ready to go on time at 7:30.

She was 42 years of age, a wife and the mother of two adolescent sons. She was also a police officer. She was controlled, stoic, cracking jokes, and answered all my admitting questions with accuracy. Mrs. Jones was a model of courage, and she also had a huge tumor in her left lung. Her prognosis depended on what and how big the tumor really was. Her husband was at her side, and I could sense he was a bit nervous, but he put on a great show as a support to her.

After the anesthesiologist finished going over the procedure for epidural anesthesia administration and had her sign consent, he asked that her husband "step out" so he could start to insert lines, along with other steps. We gave them a few moments of privacy and she seemed to be doing well after he left. I popped my head in a few times during epidural insertion and she was comfortable, cooperating well, and insertion was going along nicely. Things with my patients were going smoothly, and I would get them all ready on time with no problem.

After the epidural catheter was secured in place, I helped Mrs. Jones get back onto the stretcher. Her surgeon came down and went over the procedure with her, and asked if she had any questions. They discussed time frame issues, and I was impressed with her preparedness and knowledge of the situation. It was then 7:20 and we were ready to get her into the operating room by 7:30. Success! The benchmarkers will be proud! Epidural insertion and still on time!

As I was getting ready to say, "Good luck and God bless," Mrs. Jones grabbed my hand. She looked me in the eyes and said, "Please tell me that he's a good surgeon. I really don't care about myself, but I have two young boys and I want them to have their mother to raise them. My husband is a great father, but I'm their mother. I need to know that I made a good choice." With that, she started to cry and lowered her head. I was just about to talk to her about how I truly felt she was blessed to have the team she did taking care of her when someone called my name. "Grayce, I have a type and screen that needs to go." Mrs. Jones looked at me and said, " I'm so sorry, I'm keeping you from your work. I know you're busy. I'll be OK."

I poked my head out of the curtains, flagged a colleague to deal with the type and screen, saw the benchmarker standing there with his pen and clipboard, told the anesthesiologist that I needed five minutes, and went back inside to Mrs. Jones. I then said, "Kelly, you're not keeping me from doing my job, this *is* my job."

For five minutes, we talked and cried as she let go of her composure and was allowed to face her fear. I told her that the surgeon she picked would have been my choice and that her anesthesiologist was a staff favorite, noted for his skill and judgment. I explained that I really felt there was a good karma around her and that everything was really progressing nicely. We then talked as two mothers who love our children above anything else. We talked about how the fear of not being there for them must be universal among all mothers. I looked at this woman and knew I would be feeling the same in her position. She then told me that no matter what happened, she felt she had already left her mark on her boys and they would never forget her. They would be OK with their father and extended family. I asked her to try to concentrate on seeing the boys after surgery and to deal with issues one at a time. I reinforced that she should also remember that there was just as good a chance that she would grow old and be a burden to those boys someday. I asked her to close her eyes and picture herself reading bedtime stories to her grandchildren.

We hugged for a few minutes and then she said, "Thank you Grayce, I feel so much better. You're a really good nurse." I thanked Mrs. Jones and took the brake off the stretcher. The anesthesiologist came around the curtain and asked if we were ready to go. Mrs. Jones answered "Yes" with a smile at me. I helped them to the door and whispered, "Good luck and God bless" with a kiss to the forehead and a squeeze of the hand. "Keep good thoughts," I said as we parted ways. Mrs. Jones was smiling as she was being wheeled to the OR. It was 7:35.

The benchmarker asked me why there was a delay in departure. I told him that I needed the extra five minutes to be nurse.

CHAPTER 27

I MADE A DIFFERENCE

BY HEATHER TOMLINSON LEVY

My story focuses on an incident that occurred as I was working in the ambulatory care clinic. As part of the vascular surgery outpatient clinic, the indigent patient population was treated for venous stasis ulcers in the unna boot clinic. This clinic was held on Wednesday mornings from 6:30 am to 9:00 am. We typically had an average of twenty patients in this short span of time.

Mr. Foster was a 58-year-old African-American. He was well known to me as a regular patient. Seven years earlier, he had his right leg amputated below the knee because his circulation was very bad. He came to us with severe ulcers on his left leg. The doctors recommended amputation of this leg many times, but Mr. Foster refused the intervention. "I'd rather be with God than lose my leg. I'd have no independence without it," he'd say. Therefore, the only other treatment option was a special boot that supports the leg and encourages blood to return from it. His leg was very swollen and the ulcer was draining so badly that the dressing was constantly soaked. The skin was very damaged and the leg had a foul odor. But he was always jovial, smiling with a toothless grin, seemingly oblivious to the severity of his condition. He faithfully kept his appointments at the clinic.

One day, Mr. Foster arrived via Tele-ride, the local bus service, at 6:30 am because he was in a wheel chair. There was only one patient care technician with me in the clinic, but fortunately, no other patients had arrived. Upon entering Mr. Foster's room, I immediately noticed his eyes. They seemed sunken and had dark circles beneath them. Then I noticed the smell. It was not the same wound odor—this was stronger. As the technician and I knelt down to remove his dressing, I noticed feces on his pant leg. Before I could question him, he told me he was feeling sick and had gone to the emergency room four days earlier for a stomach ache and diarrhea. I asked if they gave him any medicine. He had received a prescription, but didn't fill it because his Social Security check had not come. He was going to go to the hospital pharmacy after his dressing change to get his medication at a discount. As we took the dressing down, I noticed the feces had actually gotten into his dressing and was on the wound. His leg was now even more damaged than before. The skin was splitting open in several places.

As I cared for the wound, I was speaking with Mr. Foster, encouraging him to wait so the surgeon could see his leg. As he was answering me, I noticed his speech became incoherent and did not make sense. He became sluggish. I quickly checked his neurological status. I instructed the technician to get oxygen started, while I attempted to get him to respond. I was concerned with his high temperature and pulse, dangerously low blood pressure, and increasing lethargy. Although my heart was racing, I remained calm and thought clearly. I knew he needed immediate medical attention. I directed the technician to get gauze and towels. We quickly wrapped his leg as we ran to the Emergency Department. I gave the nurses a report as he was rushed into an exam room. Mr. Foster had no family and I felt an obligation to be an advocate for his wishes. I stopped the attending physician as he was exiting the room. I let him know Mr. Foster was a patient of the vascular surgery service and of his expressed wishes not to have another amputation. Knowing him as well as I did, I could hear him saying he'd rather die than lose his leg. He had refused the surgery on every visit to the clinic and it was documented multiple times. The vascular surgeon was called and confirmed what I told the ER physician— no amputation. Mr. Foster was admitted to the ICU and aggressively treated with IV antibiotics. I was relieved that his wishes were being respected even though it may not have been the most prudent course of treatment. While he was an inpatient, I came to his room every week to care for his leg. I made sure the discharge plan included a way to get his medication once discharged. He progressed rapidly, and was discharged three weeks later.

Mr. Foster returned to the clinic the week after his discharge. He was so grateful that I "helped save his leg." He made quite a fuss, and it was gratifying to know I had made such a difference. It was an even better feeling knowing I was able to take charge and handle a very stressful, life-threatening situation. It was, fortunately, a positive outcome for both of us.

CHAPTER 28

CARE AND COURAGE

BY NOEL A. KLINE

Two years ago, I worked as a staff nurse on an oncology unit at a hospital in western Maryland. My experience exposed me to the various kinds of cancer and applicable treatments. Caring for a cancer patient involves not only caring for the patient, but also their family. Cancer patients have physical, emotional, and psychological needs. A nurse who is skilled at identifying patient and family needs for emotional, physical, or psychological assistance will aid the patient and their family in early, successful recovery from illness.

I had the pleasure to know and care for Sue. She is a 27-year-old registered nurse who works in the emergency room of a regional small hospital. Sue had been a healthy, married mother of a young child before her diagnosis of breast cancer. Sue discovered cancer in her left breast after showering at home. She also complained of swelling in her left, upper arm, expressed difficulty sleeping on her chest at night, and stated she had lost her appetite, as well as weight. Sue's physician confirmed the presence of the lump in her breast and immediately sent Sue to see an oncologist. Several scans and biopsies confirmed the presence of cancer in her breast. Sue was devastated by the findings. However, she was determined to be cancer free and continue to lead a fulfilling life. Sue decided surgery was the best way to eradicate the breast cancer in the most expedient fashion.

Prior to surgery, Sue was able to take care of herself independently. Postoperatively, Sue became a person dependent upon others to meet her needs. Sue's independent nature re-appeared, however, as she learned to perform her surgical wound dressing changes and to empty blood discharge from her wound drains.

Post-operatively, Sue was drowsy, in pain, and scared. She needed support to manage her emotions and pain. The surgeon ordered a patient controlled analgesia (PCA) pump of morphine to decrease Sue's pain. The PCA works best when the patient can give him or herself pain medication by pushing a remote control switch. Sue was so drowsy post-operatively that she could not self-administer her medication. However, the PCA pump was giving her some morphine each hour. I monitored Sue's pain every hour and gave her morphine via the PCA pump as appropriate. As Sue became more aware, I instructed her on the proper use of the PCA. The first day post-op was very painful for Sue. My consistency in assessing Sue's pain did control her pain by day's end.

As Sue entered her second and third days of post-op recovery, she was feeling better and began showing signs of anxiety related to wound care. Sue at this point was out of bed and walking well. The PCA pump was still connected and she had control of her pain. Sue had a left radical mastectomy (her entire breast was removed with some of her left chest lymphatic vessels). A plastic surgeon reconstructed her left breast. The breast was a mass of tender, semi-flesh tone skin and body tissue with a scar along the lower aspect. Six drains that resembled hand grenades punctured below Sue's left side. These drains called Jackson-Pratt drains aided in the removal of excess blood from Sue's surgical wound site. Although Sue was an emergency room nurse, she had very limited experience with drains.

She had much anxiety about the drains due to the post-operative appearance of her chest. My interaction with Sue from her second post-op day through her discharge on day five was critical. I was able to effectively instruct Sue on the proper care of her wound drains, measuring the fluid output, keeping a daily record of the fluid output, and the signs and symptoms of wound infection.

I created a "shoulder bag" for Sue to carry her drains more comfortably when she walked. The "shoulder bag" was nothing more than a large Zip Lock™ bag with cotton gauze strung between the sides to act as a shoulder strap. Sue was very appreciative of the "device" and proudly wore it during her hospitalization and discharge home. My most effective intervention for Sue was my interest in her as a patient. My care helped her recover well and regain a positive self-image despite a disfigured body from surgery. Moreover, Sue had displayed courage and each day helped herself more by walking, learning wound care, and PCA pump use. Sue's husband and child greatly aided her recovery as well.

Sue's story illustrates how successful nursing care and a patient's determination in conquering a deadly disease can yield positive outcomes for not just the patient, but also the healthcare professionals involved with the patient.

The care (in the form of physical interventions) rendered by Sue's nurses and the emotional care (in the form of empathy and support) they provided helped her recover. Care and courage together are powerful!

CHAPTER 29

A PATIENT-DELIVERED EDUCATION

BY LINDA JOHNSON

Mrs. Wright, a 64-year-old patient, was diagnosed with Type II diabetes in February, 1993. She was 40 to 50 pounds overweight with multiple medical problems including high blood pressure, elevated cholesterol, congestive heart failure, a history of cardiac arrest with some brain damage, and decreased ability to walk. At the time her diabetic assessment was done, she was visibly upset with her new diagnosis and tearfully stated, "I can't do it."

Patients referred for diabetes education come with varying levels of understanding of their condition. Some are ready to begin educational activities the day of the assessment, others are not. Mrs. Wright was in the latter group. Her stress level was too high. Any attempt to educate at this point would not work.

Adding diabetes to her list of problems must have given her an overwhelming sense of loss of control. I realized that gaining her trust and beginning to restore her sense of self-control was critical to ongoing education. This would not be accomplished in one day, but the first day would set the pace.

The tension needed to be lightened. My 1990 Earth Day poster had worked well in the past and seemed to be well liked. I handed it to her. There they were the three monkeys: hear no evil, see no evil, and speak no evil. Under them was the caption, "Some things just won't go away." I had added, "But it can be managed. Diabetes is a self-managed condition. You can do it!"

Mrs. Wright smiled at it, but there was no laughter. Her eyes were still fearful. She began to talk about her health and what effect she thought diabetes would have. During this time, I closed her chart, removed my phone from the receiver, and listened. I asked only a few questions to follow up on what she was talking about. The assessment would not be completed at this appointment. Establishing a solid relationship took precedence.

Allowing her to express her fears calmed her. We then discussed my role in her care as a diabetes educator. I continued to emphasize diabetes as a self-managed condition that required proper education. I emphasized that she must be an active participant. The remainder of the time was spent with hands-on assessment of blood pressure, a fasting blood sugar, and other markers that would show how well Mrs. Wright was managing. Her blood pressure and fasting blood glucose were elevated.

I discussed my findings with her physician. Mrs. Wright's blood pressure medication was increased and we began an "oral insulin" for her diabetes. She was to return to the clinic in one week for diabetic follow-up. When walking her to the door, I felt she could really use a hug. Her return hug was tighter than mine, her eyes did water, and she said she would see me next week.

Mrs. Wright was calmer at the second appointment. Her blood pressure was lower, but her blood sugar was still high. The information I obtained at the previous appointment indicated her diabetes had been diagnosed early. I began her education with a focus on relieving fears of diabetic complications. We discussed her risk factors—steps she could take to decrease or prevent complications. I provided an overview of diabetes management. Dietary instruction remained basic with an emphasis on low fats and low concentrated sweets. Our session ended by setting short-term goals.

Mrs. Wright developed two goals to work toward over the next two weeks. The first was to follow the guidelines for the low concentrated sweets and low fat diet. The second was to keep her sugar level in the normal range. I realized that this was more of a long-term goal, but I did not ask her to change it. These decisions seemed to make her feel better.

Over the next several weeks, she received instruction in all aspects of diabetic care. During this time, we discussed her home situation. She lived with her daughter, but knew that she would be responsible for her own care. Her confidence in her ability to manage her diabetes increased with each appointment. She came with questions on most days. Mrs. Wright stated that she was not ready to monitor blood sugar at home. Financing diabetic supplies was a problem since her insurance did not cover some of her needs.

During these weeks of patient education, other problems were assessed and appropriate intervention was provided. She was referred to the social worker to review the use of her Medicaid card. A Medicaid rotation schedule was established to include the eight medications prescribed. Dietary counseling was expanded to include her heart disease. Mrs. Wright's diabetic education program also provided frequent discussions with her physician. This assisted in positive outcomes of close adherence to her regimen, decreased blood pressure, normal blood sugar, and patient satisfaction.

For a year after her diagnosis, Mrs. Wright's blood sugar remained in good control. This good control eventually came to an end in spite of her efforts. Her oral insulin was not effective any more. After discussion with her physician, another oral agent was tried. It was not successful. Her blood sugar continued to increase. She did not report any other symptoms.

I discussed insulin therapy with Mrs. Wright. In her eyes, all the fear that I had seen when she was first diagnosed with diabetes returned and with it the feeling of loss of control. She refused to accept insulin therapy and tearfully said, "I just can't stick myself."

I continued to follow-up with Mrs. Wright once a month. Her follow-up blood sugars continued to increase. She now had more symptoms, but was still adamant regarding no insulin. I decided to review the benefits of insulin therapy and reminded her how closely she would be monitored until she felt confident in her abilities. The option of being admitted to the hospital to begin the insulin treatment was offered, but she refused. She did agree to think a little more about this option, until the next appointment. A discussion with her physician did not change her mind.

For the first time, Mrs. Wright did not keep her appointment. I began to feel that I had missed something that would convince her of the importance of insulin therapy. After a day or two, I called her. She was quite sick from her diabetes and agreed to try insulin. She was scheduled for instruction in insulin preparation and administration. Education, frequent follow-up, reinforcement, and the knowledge that she had access to me or a physician 24 hours a day, 7 days a week helped to lessen her fears.

Mrs. Wright has achieved excellent control. This result was like mental medicine for her. In addition to this, she was instructed in home blood sugar monitoring. She continues to check her blood sugar two to three times per day. She is able to identify reasons for increases in her blood sugar and to remedy them. Her clinic appointments have gradually decreased to every three months. Monthly phone follow-up regarding blood sugar results remains in place. Mrs. Wright orders her own diabetic supplies and exhibits a feeling of confidence and pride in self-management.

This time spent with Mrs. Wright impressed upon me how each individual progresses at his or her own rate, and in reality, the final decision in patient care is the patient's. I feel very good about Mrs. Wright's outcome. I continue to make thorough use of the telephone when appointments are missed. I feel that Mrs. Wright knew I accepted her and her opinions, though I did not agree with her decision to delay insulin therapy.

Mrs. Wright summed it up best at one of her follow-up appointments. A church sister asked her, "Why do you do all those things like sticking your finger." Her response was, "I check my blood sugar so much because I have to know what is going on in my body and so that I feel better.

CHAPTER 30

A SPECIAL PATIENT

BY JANELLE HARRIS

Mr. Finley was just one of those patients for me. The kind you hold a special relationship with from the time of admission. He was admitted with skin cancer on his left temple and was to have surgery. This turned into a six-month hospital stay when the cancer was found to involve the underlying bone, requiring major surgical reconstruction. Therapy then involved six weeks of radiation treatment. As the six months unfolded, I realized how hard it was on Mr. Finley, as day in and day out, he tolerated our routine. Who wouldn't get tired of vital signs three times a day, even though they haven't changed in weeks? Or of nurses on all three shifts asking him the same questions over and over?

Sensing his discomfort, I tried to sit with him and talk about topics unrelated to his surgery or the hospital environment. I can remember just listening to him talk about what he used to do for a living, feeling his sense of pride as he spoke of life outside the hospital. I also found out something very interesting about this well-educated lawyer. He was homeless, living on the streets of San Francisco. I found that through an unfortunate set of circumstances, he now found himself without a home and without family or resources to end this lifestyle. Throughout his hospital stay I worked with Mr. Finley and the social worker to prepare for his discharge. I checked with the social worker on a regular basis to see what discharge plans had been arranged for Mr. Finley. The social worker assured me she was still working on them. As I spoke with Mr. Finley he shared with me his hopes of once again finding a job and starting over away from the streets.

The big day of discharge finally arrived for Mr. Finley. I had been off for two days and was packing his bag to leave. I remember going into his room to find out what the discharge plans were. I could sense Mr. Finley's hopelessness as I walked into his room and saw him packing all of his belongings into a single bag. By the expression on his face, I knew the news was not good. I asked him where he was going when he left the hospital, and his answer is still clear in my mind. He told me the social worker had found him a hotel to stay in (in one of the worst sections of San Francisco). When I asked him for how long, he said, "for seven." I replied, "For seven weeks?" "Oh no, for seven days," he replied. Then I asked him what he would do after the seven days were up. He said he would return to the streets. He also reiterated that he did not want to go back to the streets, but had no other resources.

Mr. Finley had become a very special patient to me and his sense of despair urged me to find another option. I had learned early in my career that caring for a patient doesn't end at the hospital door, but includes discharge planning. Discharge planning includes enhancing the patient's ability to maintain health. Mr. Finley could have been smoothly discharged to the hotel, but I felt my responsibility went beyond getting him out of the hospital. I knew there had to be a better option.

I knew of a program that assisted homeless people who were willing to work at getting off the street. They provided living quarters, food, and a scheduled program that helped them find a job. I told Mr. Finley that I would do all I could to keep him off the streets. I told him about the program and asked if he would be interested in it. Immediately, hope returned to Mr. Finley's eyes. I made a call to the program. They had two places available. I provided Mr. Finley with the program's phone number and necessary information to get signed up. Within a matter of 30 minutes, Mr. Finley went from hopeless to a man with a new lease on life. Mr. Finley would join the program within a week. I left the hospital that day with a sense of satisfaction and joy. I was pleased I got involved with Mr. Finley and was able to do something for him that will affect the rest of his life.

I saw Mr. Finley about two months after his discharge. His face was still beaming. He expressed his thankfulness to me for caring enough to find the program that gave him hope. He is so grateful to have a bed to sleep in, food to eat, and most importantly, purpose and meaning to his life. The program is providing the resources to get his life in order. Every time I see Mr. Finley he thanks me. I know Mr. Finley will never know I am just as thankful to be part of the nursing profession that gives me the opportunity to make life-changing differences in patents' lives every day.

CHAPTER 31

A SPECIAL PLACE IN MY HEART

BY KELLY A. CAVINS

I'm very thankful today as I sit here on this beautiful Easter Sunday at Colonial Lake. I'm thankful for my two good legs that have allowed me to walk around the lake. My patient, Mrs. Dodd, isn't as fortunate as myself. She was admitted to our ward from her home in Hilton Head to rule out multiple sclerosis. Upon admission she stated, "My legs just keep getting weaker and now I can't walk." Mrs. Dodd also presented with an unexplained weight loss of 80 pounds, anorexia, night sweats, and fevers. We ruled out multiple sclerosis, but diagnosed her as having AIDS. She unfortunately had a brief sexual relation with a man whom she later discovered was an IV drug abuser.

I'll never forget the day Dr. King, the attending physician, requested a female nurse to accompany him down the hall. I readily agreed. On our way to Room 713 he informed me that we were going to tell Mrs. Dodd that she has AIDS. My heart dropped to my stomach.

Drs. King and Sipes informed her of her diagnosis with great compassion and concern. After spending some time with her, they left. There sat Mrs. Dodd and I looking at each other with tears in our eyes. I went to her and just started hugging her. She was in shock and kept repeating, "I can't believe this." It was a beautiful sunny day so we decided to go outside for some fresh air and for a change of scenery. We got her all packed up in her wheelchair complete with her soda and cigarettes. At this point my shift was over, but there was no way I was going to leave her all alone. All of her family and friends were out of town. I was the one person she could confide in at this time. We found a nice, sunny, secluded place outside where we talked, cried, laughed, and really got to know each other. She asked me, "Is this your specialty job, counseling people with AIDS?" I had to admit to her that this was my first experience. She then stated, "You're so good at it, I thought you did it all the time."

Mrs. Dodd and I have become friends through this tragic period in her life. She was started on medication and intense physical therapy. She is now able to walk some on her own, though her wheelchair remains close by. Mrs. Dodd always comes to visit when she is at the hospital for her follow-up appointments. At present she is doing well physically and has become an active member of an AIDS support group.

Mrs. Dodd will always hold a special place in my heart and I'm sure I'll be in hers.

CHAPTER 32

THE ART OF NURSING

BY DEBORAH J. DOWNES

I was about to start my third, twelve-hour night shift for the week. Perpetually exhausted, I took a deep breath and whispered a silent prayer before looking at my assignment. My heart sank when I saw that Mrs. Fry was to be one of my patients. Difficult patients were always rotated among the staff, in a half-hearted attempt by the charge nurse to prevent burn-out. I wanted to cry and run screaming from the building. But why should this night be different from any other? It was bad enough that I always had more patients than I could effectively care for (let alone chart on), but this one patient was every nurse's nightmare: virtually full-care, fully conscious, and with a bad attitude. She had been in a terrible car crash, in which she had suffered multiple broken bones and contusions. Worse yet, she was understandably in severe pain, and *not* on patient-controlled anesthesia. This would increase my paperwork, and send me running for the pain medications every four hours.

I took another deep breath and said another prayer (God is my copilot) before entering the room to assess her. I was prepared for the usual harangue of complaints about the care. I was dealing with the "five toos" of nursing: too many patients, too little help, too much documentation, too many medications, and too much stress! I was therefore very surprised to find her quietly crying and looking quite pathetic, amid a prison of wires, tubing, splints, and bed rails, which prevented her from moving in any purposeful way. She was black and blue wherever skin was visible. Her once well-coifed hair was matted, and the smells of neglect could not be masked by her expensive perfume. She had been hospitalized for at least a week, and it certainly appeared that she had had little in the way of personal care. Even through this mess, I could see that she had probably been attractive, well-groomed, and of the sort who regularly had her hair and nails done (the remnants of an expensive manicure were still in evidence).

I had been prepared to do battle, only to find that my adversary was more helpless than a sick child. As a seasoned nurse, I had become inured to many things in an effort to get the job done. After all, calm, cool, and collected was the only way to maintain professionalism and competency in a health care system run amok, right? But therein lies the paradox of nursing, that we, who are drawn to this profession because of a need to give compassionate care, are nevertheless expected to remain objectively aloof, and even militaristic in our approach to patient care. Be that as it may, my resolve was washed away by her tears, and helping this poor lady to feel better became my priority for the shift. Documentation be damned!

I administered her medications, and made her as comfortable as I could, for the moment. Then I assured her that I would be back to spend some quality time with her, just as soon as I had completed my rounds. She nodded forlornly, though I am sure that she did not believe me, as I could not believe that she was the same person who had been giving the staff such a hard time. Later, I learned that she had given up hope, all together.

I did return, as promised, with one of our two nursing assistants (this was a 30-bed unit), and an armload of clean linen and bathing supplies, all of which were very difficult to conjure up on the night shift. We then took the time to clean her thoroughly and gently, while conversing with her, all the while. I tried to employ the techniques for therapeutic communication that I had learned back in nursing school, and had not used since. It wasn't difficult, since she did most of the talking. The car crash that had nearly killed her was, in fact, the least of her troubles. Several years earlier, she had lost her daughter in a freak accident. More recently, she had battled breast cancer and the loss of her husband. She was just starting to get back on track, when this accident occurred.

She freely admitted to being hard to please and demanding, but she had never felt so helpless or hopeless before. Not surprisingly, she also confessed that her mental agony far outweighed her physical pain. Although a wealthy woman who could afford to indulge any whim, she had been unable to compensate for the love she had lost. Now she had lost the last shreds of her dignity and self-esteem. Nothing more could be taken from her. I was overwhelmed with sadness for her, and I realized that, although I could not reverse her tragedies, I had at least restored her dignity and self-worth to some degree.

The gratitude that she expressed to us was so sincere, that I still get misty-eyed when I think of her. What never ceases to amaze me, is the fact that, in reality, what I had done was so simple and so basic. I had touched her body with caring hands, and touched her spirit with caring words and a willingness to listen; and she had, likewise, touched me.

For better or worse, no one else had shared our bond. It is nowhere legally documented; it is not a billable item, nor subject to pre-approval by an insurance company, nor described under hospital policy and procedure. Yet it clarifies the reason why I chose to become a nurse, and for me, it is the heart and soul of nursing—namely, that priceless and curative connection between a nurse and her patient, which leaves both feeling valued. It is a feeling that once experienced, becomes addictive. How inordinately tragic that it cannot be validated by research, or quantified by the auditors! Yet without it, nursing is merely a mundane job instead of an artistic profession.

CHAPTER 33

A FINAL SMILE

BY MARIE DANIEL

Brother Walter has scleroderma, a disease that affects most body organs. It is progressive and there is no known cure. His disease continued to progress and affect his lungs and heart. His stamina and energy were waning, requiring the monastery physicians to accompany him on frequent visits to the clinic. He also endured several hospital admissions. Ultimately, portable oxygen tanks became his constant companions. With these additional burdens, and his physical compromise, Brother Walter still carried a smile, his sense of humor, his beautiful humility, and acceptance of his fate.

One morning, Brother Walter was having increasing difficulty breathing. He was on his supplemental oxygen, but was obviously deteriorating and his physician was called. In order to evaluate his condition, Brother Walter was scheduled to see his cardiologist that afternoon. I was looking forward to the end of a long day, when I saw Brother Walter in the waiting room. Noting his difficulty breathing and what we as nurses have learned to trust as a sixth sense, I knew something wasn't right. He was obviously in more respiratory distress than usual, and he no longer greeted me with his bright smile.

I immediately took over his visit and called the physician to report my feelings. The physician asked for a measure of his oxygen saturation with and without his supplemental oxygen. I proceeded with this testing and his oxygen saturation was only 87%. I reported this information back to the physician over the telephone, who then told me to turn his oxygen from his current 3 liters, to 5 liters, and send the patient home. Having worked with Brother Walter for many months, I sensed in him a fear and somewhat reserved panic. Though medically appropriate, I felt that to send Brother Walter away to the monastery with increased oxygen might support his physical needs, but at this stage of his disease, I felt he needed something more. Never being one to second-guess or question a physician's decision, I instructed Brother Walter's companion to bring the car to the hospital entrance to eliminate Brother Walter's exposure to the cold. As Brother Walter and I waited for his companion, we talked a bit more about his condition. Knowing how trusting he was of his health care providers and his uncomplaining manner, I knew that if he had concerns, they would go unspoken. It concerned me that his usual good humor and positive attitude had been replaced with an unusual complacency. It was at this time that I too began to feel a reserved panic.

As we waited for the elevator to take Brother Walter to the hospital entrance and his awaiting companion, I found myself torn between sending him from a very secure safe environment and following the physician's orders or turning back and calling the physician once again. Over the years I have learned that following my gut instinct and listening to patients with my eyes and ears is usually the most appropriate decision. I was seeing not only the medical numbers—both oxygen liters and oxygen saturation—but also a man that was demonstrating unspoken signs of physical distress and emotional turmoil. Brother Walter had become such a frequent patient in the clinic that I knew he trusted us with his well-being and treatment. I felt to send him away would betray that trust as well as my instinct that I have learned to trust. Rather than ignore my feelings, I chose to call the physician and again stress my concerns. It was at that moment that I turned the oxygen up to its maximum flow, and returned to the clinic. With his condition deteriorating as it was, he needed to be in a setting where technology was minutes and not hours away.

Once in the clinic, I rechecked his oxygen saturation, and found my instincts had been correct. Even administering more oxygen than I had been ordered to send him home on, his oxygen saturation was a mere 82%. It was now after 5:00 PM and most of the clinic staff had left for the day. I asked one of the remaining staff members who was on her way out to please notify Brother Walter's companion that we were very possibly going to admit Brother Walter. I found myself alone with Brother Walter and took this time to explain to him that I felt his worsening condition warranted admission and that I wanted to speak with his physician again to ensure we were providing him with the safest care possible before sending him home. I telephoned the physician and explained emphatically that I felt Brother Walter needed to be admitted. I reported I had increased his oxygen and he had continuing decreasing oxygen saturation. I also reported my physical and emotional assessment of the patient. The physician reluctantly agreed and I proceeded to prepare for his admission. Knowing how the admission process works, and the length of time it requires to obtain a bed assignment, I knew that it might be quite some time before I would be able to leave Brother Walter. I left him alone only for the time it took for me to call and notify my family that I would be home quite late in the evening.

After completing his pre-admission work-up, his bed assignment was made. I transported him to his room. Even as the exhaustion of the day overcame him, he and his companion thanked me for being persistent with the physician to keep him in the hospital. They also thanked me for staying and seeing him through the admission. Being in a teaching institution, I remained the only constant in Brother Walter's treatment. By helping him make the transition from outpatient to an inpatient, I knew my presence there had a familiar calming effect.

Brother Walter's companion had to leave to return to the monastery. Though it had also been a long day for me, I did not want to leave Brother Walter alone. I sat with him and we discussed his disease and his prognosis. He told me that his fears were not about death, but the act of dying. He was concerned about his increasing struggle to breathe and his feelings of suffocation. Even facing these fears and discussing them with me, he was quick to assure me that his trust in God was complete and that he would handle whatever he had to face with God's help. I was touched by our conversation as he talked about his total acceptance of God's will, because his feelings so closely parallel mine. I stayed almost an hour with him that evening and left wishing I could have stayed longer.

I realized as I left that discussing his spirituality had helped to reinforce my faith and helped resolve my earlier questions of how God could let something like this happen to a man who had so obviously dedicated his life to him. Brother Walter was living the disease and didn't question it. Just as I was his nurse and shouldn't question my instinct for what is right. Brother Walter's strength and faith touched me and left me with such a peaceful feeling. I saw Brother Walter face his life and disease with such faith, dedication, and conviction, that I knew I would never again betray my own instinct of what is the most appropriate care for a patient.

I am devoted to my patients and my career as a nurse, just as Brother Walter is devoted to the church and his life as a monk. I will now face my nursing instincts with the same faith, dedication, and conviction. I know that never again will I ignore those instincts for fear of physician disapproval. Taking a risk, and questioning a physician's judgement turned out to be best for Brother Walter and also signified a turning point in my nursing career. I feel that as a health care team, we are just that, a health care team. My chosen profession of nursing is not just providing medical care and following physician orders, but rather treating the patient as a whole. To provide excellent care requires incorporating the physical, spiritual, and emotional aspects of the person. Brother Walter was my patient, but also a person with fears and concerns that needed to be addressed.

As Brother Walter's condition worsened, he was discharged back to the monastery and the decision was made to forego further treatment. Hospice became involved in his care, and I no longer had the opportunity to experience his smiling face on a weekly basis. I continued to check with his physicians on his condition, and frequently called the monastery to check on him. I soon learned that his family had traveled to be with him, and though I yearned to visit him again in what I knew were his final days, I did not want to intrude. In early August I took several days off, and though it had been six months since I had seen him, my thoughts were of him often. I decided to visit Brother Walter at the monastery, but ironically upon calling the monastery on the day I had intended to visit, I learned that Brother Walter had passed away. I decided that I would proceed with my visit and attend his funeral.

I arrived at the funeral and met Father Gallagher. He told me of how much Brother Walter thought of me and how grateful he was for my concern and care. He took me to meet some of the other monks, and to my surprise they all knew who I was. It seems that Brother Walter had been so touched by our relationship that he had told them all about me. I was so touched hearing them talk of Brother Walter and his words about me, that I began to cry. They told me that he had died a peaceful death and that at the moment of his death, a smile appeared on his face. From our conversation on the night of his admission, I knew that he had not been afraid of death, but of the act of dying. It brought me great peace to know that he had not suffered in his act of dying. I will always be grateful to have had the opportunity to know and work with such a holy man, and I will continue to follow my instincts that have been formed from my many years of truly listening to and assessing my patients. I have noticed that my compassion and empathy for my patients has increased greatly since my experience with Brother Walter. I seem to be able to deal with my patients and their chronic and often terminal illnesses with better understanding and more open communication. I also have a deeper appreciation for the need of terminal patients to have the support of family, friends, and their caretakers, to help them face death. Though Brother Walter's true family was not with him for the majority of his illness, his real family was his monastery family. Possessing a deep faith in God also helps when facing a terminal illness. Though many are not comfortable talking of spirituality with their health care providers, I now try to incorporate an assessment of a patient's spirituality and beliefs. For patients like Brother Walter, with whom spirituality is a crucial element to facing the end of life, I know that taking the time to talk with them will enhance *my* relationship with them.

CHAPTER 34

A LESSON IN TOTAL PATIENT CARE

BY ANN E. MARSH

Our emergency department was busy when we received a radio call from a local ambulance company late one afternoon. The caller informed us there had been a one-vehicle rollover crash. One occupant was thrown clear of the car; the other occupant needed to be extricated by the Fire Department. Both patients were arriving fully immobilized. We were also instructed that Medflight, the medical helicopter service, already had been activated and would be arriving soon at the emergency department.

Upon arrival of the patients, we learned they were husband and wife. Since the emergency room was already full, it was not possible to place them in the same room. The wife was sent to the acute care area where the staff continued to assess her and to prepare her for flight to a trauma center. The patient was alert, oriented, tearful, and distraught about the condition her husband. The staff reassured her often, promising to get her information about her husband as soon as possible.

The husband was more stable and sent to the treatment area. As his assessment continued, he was equally concerned about his wife's condition. Again the staff assured him they would get him information as soon as possible.

When the physician informed the husband of his wife's condition, and that she would be transferred to a trauma center, the husband naturally asked to see her before she left. When the physician told the nurse of the husband's request, and asked if it would be possible, the nurse replied, "of course." The patient was cautioned that although we would gladly take him to his wife, both of them had to remain immobile.

The husband was wheeled into his wife's room, their stretchers placed parallel with one another, as the nursing staff quietly worked around them, preparing her for her flight. We found the sight not only touching, but slightly amusing. There they lay, both immobilized, staring at the ceiling, but with fingers intertwined, talking of the recent events. The wife suddenly said, "where's the baby?" The nursing staff feared the worst. Had an infant gone unnoticed at the scene? We questioned them about the baby. They tearfully explained there was a three-month old dachshund puppy in the car with them. While relieved this was not a human infant, we began to worry about the pup that was so precious to our patients. We assured them we would do whatever we could to locate the puppy.

Martie, one of the staff, called the ambulance service that had delivered our patients. They said yes, there had been a dog on the scene. They said the dog was taken to the local fire station for safety, until someone claimed it. Wanda called the fire station and verified they had the dog. The also said they had no one available to bring the dog to the hospital. Wanda, the nurse, then called her son Charles who was visiting his girlfriend in the area. Charles agreed to go pick up the puppy. At this point, Martie and Wanda thought it might be a good idea to inform Betsy, the charge nurse, of their activities. Wanda told Betsy that her son was bringing the dog to the emergency room, as asked, "Is that OK?" Betsy assured her that it was, asking to be informed when the guest arrived.

Medflight arrived, efficiently prepared the wife for transport, and departed. The husband had been taken upstairs to have a scan of his abdomen. Charles and his girlfriend Brittany appeared at the employee entrance with a very small, very scared puppy. The puppy was wrapped in a white blanket, her big brown eyes looking around nervously as she shivered in anxiety. Betsy took the puppy from Charles and held her close, whispering soft words into her ear. We all went to the family room. As we are avid animal lovers, it was important to know the puppy was not hurt. When we placed her on the floor, she immediately fell to her right, her front shoulder was unable to bear weight. We examined the leg carefully. While we couldn't find any obvious injury, we knew that we were a bit unsure of normal bone structure in dachshunds. We carefully splinted the leg as a precaution.

Christy, one of the x-ray technicians, showed up, curious about the commotion. As I held the pup in my arms, I smiled at her and asked, "Feel like x-raying something unusual?" She quickly agreed, telling us she had x-rayed the hip of a German Shepherd once for a local physician. As I held the puppy in position, Christ shot the x-ray. We waited in the back hallway for the pup's owner to return from his x-ray. As the puppy continued to shake, Charles told us of how frightened she became when he started his car. Betsy reminded him that the pup's last car trip was pretty traumatic.

At this moment, the owner returned. What a thrill it was to be able to place that little dog in her owner's arms. He gathered her up quickly. She snuggled close to him just as quickly. It was so obvious this reunion was the best medicine for both of them. He told us her name was Sissy. Our medical director, Dr. Bill, happened by at that time. We showed him the x-ray, and he examined Sissy's leg. While he reminded the owner that he wasn't a veterinarian, he felt her injury was a short-term nerve trauma, one that she would recover from easily. Dr. Bill advised a trip to their vet in the near future. As we started back to the treatment area, Christy handed us a copy of Sissy's x-ray so the owner could take it the vet with him.

We wheeled both of our patients back to the treatment room; Sissy nestled in her owner's arms. The owner asked Betsy if he could go out to smoke, stating that he felt really nervous. Betsy cautioned that we needed his x-ray result before that was a good idea. She suggested he stay with Sissy, calming her. Betsy turned the lights down, and quietly left the room.

As it was shift change, Betsy gave a report to her counterpart from the night shift. She took her to room 11 to introduce her to the new patient, and to let the husband know she was leaving for the day. While it had only been minutes since the man needed a smoke for his shaken nerves, when Betsy peeked into the room, the husband was sound asleep, snoring softly. Sissy was tucked in the crook of his arm, her long nose resting on his chest. Sissy opened her eyes when she heard Betsy, then promptly went back to sleep.

Words cannot describe the effect this family and reunion had on us. It impressed upon us once again that total patient care sometimes means looking beyond the patient in front of you. Sometimes it means listening closely to the patient and reaching outside of your comfort zone.

CHAPTER 35

OOPS

BY KATHY CASTILLE-ALIFFI

Intensive care can be a very stressful and rewarding environment for any nurse, and it is really the experiences that we share that helps us bond and grow together while we work to save lives and heal patients. This is one special moment between two nurses that will endure in our memories for years to come, perhaps for our lifetime. One uneventful day another nurse, Patty, and myself were sitting in the ICU nurses station writing notes in the patients' charts. We could both see an older gentleman visitor at the beside of a patient. As he stood in the room he had his hat in his hand, praying perhaps, or merely observing the patient who was unconscious and on life support (ventilator). After a few moments he came out of the room and walked to where we were seated.

The man quietly asked us "What is the bottom line?" Patty and I looked at each other knowing that this question and the conversation will be one of hopelessness for this gentleman. I replied "Well, the bottom line is that he isn't doing very well. His case is very complicated and so much is being done for him. It's really hard to tell what is going to happen. It doesn't look good." He held his hat and replied softly "I know, but what is the bottom line?" At this point Patty and I looked at one another again, for it's always difficult when either of us has to tell a family member that the patient is dying.

Patty replied this time, "Well, he isn't doing very well. His lab work is abnormal and he still isn't breathing on his own. I don't think he is going to make it considering the problems and his age. We just don't know, really." At this point the gentleman who was wringing his hat in his hands said more assertively, "I understand all that. I just want to know what's that bottom line!"

as he pointed his finger at the cardiac monitor display on the wall of the patients room. Patty and I looked at each other once again, eyes wide open, and responded in unison "Oh, *that* bottom line!"

This gentleman wanted to know more about the waveforms on the monitor and what the information is used for. We were so consumed with the need to break the news to this nice quiet man as gently as possible that we didn't realize that perhaps he wanted something else. So to this day, that one shared moment has bonded the two of us together and when I see Patty I always ask her, "Hey! What's the bottom line?"

CHAPTER 36

A DAY TO REMEMBER

BY MELODY C. ANTOON

During my career as a registered nurse, I have encountered many situations that have made me look at the world, society, and most importantly, myself, differently. I have come to look at illness, poverty, conflict, family, and lifestyles with an empathetic, open, and non-judgmental attitude as compared to my pre-nursing views.

As a home health nurse, I cared for people from many walks of life. Caring for a patient in their own home is quite different than providing that same care in a hospital setting. In many situations, the home health nurse becomes a part of the family. The impact of the illness on the family and the patient in their "real life" surroundings can be an eye-opening experience.

There are many situations and families that were special to me as a home health nurse, but one family in particular stands out in my mind. Ms. Ann was in her late 50s. She lived with her son, Bo, who was probably in his late 20s but functioned at a third grade level. On my first visit to their home, I filled out the usual paper work which included a list of her medications, her vital signs, and her diagnosis. Ms. Ann had diabetes and, as a result, had very poor vision. I noticed that she had no shoes on and was dressed in tattered clothing. Bo stayed outside working on an old Ford that was not running at the time. It was their only form of transportation. The tiny house trailer was clean, but old and not air conditioned. In South Louisiana and in the middle of the summer, the heat can be stifling; not to mention the flies. She fanned herself as I did my assessment and asked questions. A tall glass of iced tea sounded wonderful but I declined her offer. I decided to wait for something to drink after I left her house. I finished my assessment, obtained her signatures (an "X"), and quickly went to the comfort of my air conditioned vehicle and the next home visit in a lovely, cool home. I felt fortunate that the majority of my patients lived in homes where I felt comfortable.

For the first two weeks, I saw Ms. Ann three times a week. Her blood sugar was not stable. My suspicion was that she was not taking her medications as directed by her doctor. I obtained a pill box and I personally filled it for her hoping that would solve the problem. It did seem to get better and her blood sugar levels became more stable. At that point, I decided to see her only once a week. However, as I was filling her pill box and telling her that I would only be coming once a week now instead of three times a week, her medications ran out. I was unable to fill the pill box for the entire week. There was no medication for the last four days of the week. I told Ms. Ann to have Bo go to the pharmacy and refill her prescriptions. Then I would come back and finish filling her pill box. At that point, she looked at the floor and, almost in a whisper, told me that they had no money to refill her medications for that month. Finally, I realized why her blood sugar had been so hard to control. She could not afford to pay for the medicine. I used my cell phone (they did not have telephone service) to call doctors' offices to find samples to get her through the month. She would be able to fill her prescriptions at the beginning of next month. The crisis was over; or so I thought.

The next month rolled around and I was relieved to be successful at getting Ms. Ann on a once weekly schedule. Each week I went to see her, I would stay a little longer than the previous visit. I was beginning to develop a relationship with this woman and her son. They would share stories with me of their past and I would listen. I always sat in a large antique rocker that was the only comfortable chair in the house. It was also, in my opinion, a lovely antique! I had never seen claw feet on a rocker before. When I mentioned it to Ms. Ann, she told me that they had picked it up from a discard pile on the side of the road. They needed a chair and it was free. Every time I would come to visit, I would sit in that rocker and drink a glass of iced tea with Ms. Ann and her son. I told Ms. Ann that if she ever wanted to sell the rocker, I would buy it from her. She smiled.

As the months progressed, I would end up finding Ms. Ann samples of her medication as she was never able to pay for an entire month's worth of medicine. Her diet was poor but adequate. Near the end of the month, I noticed that they had less food than at the beginning of the month. They survived on staples.

I had been seeing Ms. Ann for about six months and had become quite fond of her and her son. I looked forward to our weekly visits. They both needed dental care, and she needed new glasses. I was able to arrange transportation and free care for both of them to assist with these problems. I was beginning to feel that I was actually making a difference to this family.

On one of my visits in the dead cold of winter, I entered the chilly trailer and found Ms. Ann sitting on the sofa as usual, but looking a bit troubled. I sat down and began talking to her about her week. Was she taking her medications correctly? What was she eating? As I was writing down what she told me, she asked me a question. I did not completely hear what she said so I asked her to repeat herself. Her question to me was, "Do you still want that rocking chair?" She was talking about the chair that I was sitting in and had always admired. My response was, "Of course I would like to have the rocking chair, but I thought that you wanted to keep it?" Her reply is something I will never forget. "We need food worse than we need a rocking chair."

I had never encountered this kind of poverty in my lifetime. I went home and emptied out my refrigerator and pantry and loaded up the back of my Suburban with food to take to them. I even cooked a huge roast with rice and vegetables for them to eat that night and use the leftovers for later meals. I felt so small.

The lesson that I learned from Ms. Ann is something that changed my outlook on life. I learned the true meaning of "non-judgmental" and, in my opinion, I learned the true meaning of nursing. Nursing is truly a caring profession.

CHAPTER 37

YOU NEVER KNOW WHAT WILL HAPPEN

By Kathy Grimley Baker

Every nurse has his or her personal passionate reasons for why they went into nursing. Some are their own tragedies and others are tragedies outside of themselves. Either way, they are called to nurse.

After we finish nursing school and join our colleagues in the trenches, our patients remind us on a daily basis why we nurse. Most patient interactions inspire us and rejuvenate us, while others bring us to our knees. I know why I nurse. With more than twenty years under my stethoscope I have always felt that bedside nursing was the best. Even after getting my Masters degree in nursing, I never left the bedside, as I always felt that bedside nursing was the most fun. There is no other job that gets me as close to a person. I try to inspire my undergraduate nursing students when I teach clinical practice. Sharing the new nurse eagerness with my students is a reminder of why nursing can be powerful and important even after so many years. I had such a reminder one day while working the 3 pm–11 pm shift.

I started out with making assignments and listening to report. I assigned Mrs. A to Cathy, the other nurse working with me. The two of us always joke when we work together that the patients can't go wrong if they ask for their nurse Cathy/Kathy because that was my name also. I would also joke when staff asked for "Cathy." "Did they want the nice or evil Cathy?" I would ask. Mrs. Allen was a middle-aged woman admitted to the pain service for treatment of chronic pain from a chronic muscle disease. I heard in report that Mrs. Allen wasn't feeling well. She had complaints of nausea and had one emesis on day shift. She already had an IV, so she was stable.

Early in the shift, Cathy consulted with me about Mrs. A's complaints. Cathy went in and offered her a phenergan suppository. Mrs. Allen refused it saying, "I don't want it 'cause it really doesn't help all that much anyway." As Cathy started to leave the room, Mrs. Allen turned on her side and arched her neck back. Cathy ran to her and she wasn't responding. Cathy called me into the room. As we rolled her onto her back Mrs. Allen took a long deep breath. I was somewhat relieved. "We've got 'A' for airway," I thought. I could tell by her color that we weren't out of the woods. I shouted "Call the code team, get the crash cart."

Cathy said Mrs. Allen had a pulse but it was weak. I remember shouting at the nurse, Alice, at the crash cart "I can't find the 'on' switch." Alice put it on. As little as I knew about EKGs, I knew we were in trouble. I checked for a pulse and I swear I felt nothing. I grabbed someone's stethoscope off their neck and placed it on Mrs. A's chest. I couldn't believe the silence. I heard nothing. Oh wait, she is breathing. So we've got A (airway), B (breathing), but no C (circulation). I shouted "I am starting chest compressions." "One and two and three and four and five." I could feel my voice cracking as I thought to myself, God why are you making me do this? My emotions were starting to take over. To keep myself together I shouted louder "one and two and three and four and five!" repeating the mantra until the code team arrived. At the time when I was doing chest compressions I couldn't help thinking about how the nurses on the 3–11 shift used to joke that years from now, when we were old and gray, we would get a big, black, circular tattoo on the center of the chest that would say "DON'T PUSH HERE."

The code team arrived. The doctor said "I want to know the story on this patient." Someone shouted, "She is Cathy's patient." He saw my nametag with 'Kathy' and looked at me. It was almost funny when I said to the rhythm of my counting, "You want Cathy P not Kathy GB." The electrocardiogram was flat, meaning the heart was not pumping blood. The code team shocked her and got her rhythm back. They put an IV into her leg and a tube into her lungs to aid in breathing, and off we went to the intensive care unit. I thought that one of the nurses from the code team looked slightly familiar but with all the chaos I didn't give it a second thought. When I arrived at the intensive care unit, one of my favorite nurses, Cookie, from when I was a new graduate was there to greet me and the patient. Cookie asked, "You still work here?" My response was "Yeah, it happens to the best of us. Some folks will do anything for a free parking permit for thirty years of service."

I continued to take notes on the clipboard. Things were calming down and the baton was slowly being turned over to the intensive care unit staff. I looked more closely at the blonde pony-tailed nurse from the code team. 'Oh my gosh,' I thought. She looked a lot like a student from my senior leadership course at the University of San Francisco ten years ago. Then, as I heard staff talking to her, it confirmed who she was. As I was about to go back to my nice quiet floor, I placed my hand on Katie's shoulder and said "I taught you ten years ago in senior leadership." Katie was shocked, but did remember me.

Upon returning to my unit, I was asked by staff (especially Lynn) if I had followed up on Mrs. Allen's condition. I gave the usual professional answer that with the new confidentiality regulations she was no longer our patient and her condition was no longer any of our business. The reality was, emotionally, I could not handle the news if it wasn't good.

Almost a week went by and I was back at work. I walked down the hall and started making the assignment when my nurse Lynn asked, "Did you see Mrs. Allen?" I didn't know what she was talking about. Then she informed me I had walked right passed Mrs. Allen when I came on the unit. She was the one with the IV pole walking in the hall. I didn't even recognize her. It is amazing what a pumping heart can do for someone's color! As staff starting coming in for report they thought I should take her since I was the one that did CPR on her. I started to get emotional explaining how blown away I was. I would go and visit her later.

I took some time after report to check on my patients and get myself together to see her. When I walked into her room, someone from physical therapy was there. I touched Mrs. Allen's arm and told her I couldn't believe she was here. I told her I just wanted to look at her for a moment. Mrs. Allen said, "They said you were here. You are the one that saved my life." I touched her face on the side up by her forehead and told her I was so glad she was alive and healthy. Her response as I headed out of the room was a shout that she was glad to be back with the living! She was scheduled for a pacemaker later that week.

It isn't often that we as nurses actually save lives so dramatically. For some reason, I guess it was my turn. I didn't sign up for it. But it is nice to know that I did rise to the occasion. I hope this takes care of me for my next decade. I still want that free parking permit.

CHAPTER 38

THE FIRST TIME I SAW GRACE

BY PENNIE DEBOARD

The first time I saw Grace, her silver hair and bent frame told of someone well into their eighth decade of life. In the handful of months after our first encounter, this patient would surprise and enlighten me many times. She would also steal my heart and gift me with the human side to my profession.

Grace suffered from psoriasis for many years, but it was after the ravaging effects of a terminal respiratory disease, and the reoccurrence of breast cancer, that she began to have difficulty controlling her now ever-worsening skin condition. In hopes of relief, Grace came to see one of the physicians in the large dermatology clinic where I worked.

As a staff nurse at the clinic, I had treated many patients who had psoriasis, and knew how much difference a supportive family member made in the patient's well being. Nevertheless, I was always touched by how gentle and considerate Grace's husband was during her office visits.

Murmuring softly to her as he worked, he would carefully assist in the undressing that was necessary for her examination. I was young, and at first attempted to intervene, feeling that it should be "my job" to help the patient disrobe. Over time, however, I came to understand that it was therapeutic for them both, and instead folded and set aside her garments as they were removed.

It was during these few minutes that Grace and I would converse—initially about her treatments and medications, and later, when we knew each other better, about children and flower gardens. When the creams and ointments prescribed became ineffective, her doctor suggested she start a twice-weekly phototherapy program to quell the itching.

Grace's poor health, in combination with the heat and duration of these treatments, made it necessary to limit her time in the light box to ten minutes. As a safety factor, I stayed with her during these times, standing just outside the treatment area in case she needed assistance. To pass the time, she would share with me her feelings about special events as they unfolded in her life.

She had a grown daughter unable to have children, who would soon be adopting. The prospect of another grandchild was so exciting! Grace's husband often volunteered at the local elementary school, reading to the youngsters, and she would go too, when she felt well enough. Her sight diminished by cataracts, Grace would instead dole out hugs and a loving ear to the little ones when the teacher had her hands full.

To keep up my end of the conversation, I would share the vivid colors of my rose garden. One day, she pulled out of her pocket a recent picture of her newest granddaughter. The gesture was special because I knew I was seeing clearly with my eyes what she never would. We traded stories and laughed together. Ten minutes at a time, we had become friends.

After a few months, her worsening shortness of breath and lack of stamina forced a discontinuation of the light treatments. It became too difficult for Grace to leave her home, so her husband began an even more diligent skin care regimen, in an attempt to keep her comfortable. The patient's goals had begun to change. Grace was dying.

A few times, when I was working an evening shift at the clinic, Grace would call in, wanting to talk. Her words were clipped and she worked hard to catch her breath between them. She would update me on recent events, and listen with interest to my quick comments about the challenges of raising a family.

Later on, only her husband would phone, on the pretense of working through a treatment problem, but mostly just to talk about Grace. Like most nurses, I had two days' work to squeeze into one shift, but his calls were important to all of us and somehow I made time. Grace was doing poorly, and I was given an invitation to their home in a neighboring suburb for an informal visit. When I arrived, I found her condition worse that I expected. We talked briefly; I suggested a couple of trade tricks to make skin care easier. She surprised me with a set of bright yellow hot pads she had crocheted some months back. I didn't fail to notice that despite her blindness, each row was straight and true. Grace was a unique person and a great gift.

CHAPTER 39

AS ANGELS VISIT

BY MARCIA KECK CLINE

It was a Friday evening when I admitted Frances. She was an 88-year-old lady with a heart attack and was in shock. Her blood pressure was steadily dropping throughout the evening, despite large doses of medication. Her urine output was almost nonexistent. She was pale, cool, and clammy. Because of her request for no further means to "keep me going," we called in her family and her minister. I had requested to stay for the prayer circle around my patient. Frances seemed at peace with her decision and held out her hand to begin the prayer circle. After several prayers were said, the family stepped out of her room to talk with the minister.

After her last daughter left, Frances beckoned me to stay. Frances told me that her daughter had told her not to tell me her story as I would think she was hallucinating. But she chose to tell me that while we were praying, angels stood guard around the room. Warmth enveloped me immediately. I asked Frances if the angels were there to let her know they were ready for her. Surprisingly, Frances smiles and said, "No, they wanted me to know that they were not ready for me yet." I was surprised and thought she was hallucinating. She had no urine output or blood pressure. Her heart rate was slow and she was cold and clammy. When I left at midnight, I hugged her goodbye and told her she would be in my prayers. I was sure she would not be there the next afternoon, when I came into work.

As I strolled into work with a hazelnut latté in hand, I thought of the grey-haired lady who had been visited by angels and how she must love her new home in heaven. I walked past her room and to my surprise, there she was, smiling and waving. Frances had a normal blood pressure, urine output, heart rate, and her color was pink. She must have noticed my surprise. "I told you they weren't ready for me yet," she said happily. Frances went home a few days later.

CHAPTER 40

MAN'S BEST FRIEND

BY HELEN JUNE DANIELS

I recognized the important role pets play in health. I made a decision one day to do my own informal research study with my patient, Mr. Paree, who had just been diagnosed with terminal cancer. If anyone needed cheering up, Mr. Paree did! While my particular healthcare facility did not participate in pet therapy, I saw no harm in allowing just one, short visit from a furry, white toy French poodle by the name of Cheri.

Mr. Paree was feeling very depressed. The day before, doctors had given him very bad news: terminal cancer. At age 82, and never having been sick before, the news devastated the poor man. During my contact with Mr. Paree, I noticed a small photo of a white toy poodle tacked to the wall in front of his hospital bed. I asked about the picture and Mr. Paree beamed a response, "That's my little Cheri!"

A short time passed and my efforts to cheer up my patient were coming up short. As I stood by his bedside, the phone rang and Mr. Paree motioned for me to answer it. It was his daughter calling to see if there was anything her father needed her to bring to the hospital. "I'll be leaving for the hospital in about 15 minutes," she said. I looked at Mr. Paree's sad face, then over to the picture of his furry little pet, and I quickly said, "Yes, as a matter of fact, there *is* something, or rather, *someone* you can bring!"

Cheri Paree sat on her master's bed for the next four hours. So quiet, so tiny, yet so important was she in helping lift my patient's spirits. Her doggy kisses were just as effective as any medicine I had to offer.

The success of pet therapy hinges on this fact: pets don't care whether patients are sick, bed bound, or hooked up to machines or tubes. They simply want to love and be loved, unconditionally. Man's best friend became nurse's best friend the day a tiny little poodle worked her magic on my saddened patient. While my efforts alone to cheer up my patient fell short of the mark, the assistance of a gal named Cheri Paree proved very therapeutic in providing just what the patient needed.

CHAPTER 41

APPRECIATION OF TOUCH

BY BOZENA M. PADYKULA

When my children get tired, or cannot fall asleep, a few minutes of holding and gently massaging their hands soothes them. They fall asleep relaxed, comforted by familiar touch. I started to appreciate the value of human-to-human touch in my nursing career after my second patient fell asleep after a long and restless anxiety episode comforted by holding and gently massaging her hand. These two situations allowed me to appreciate the simple nursing intervention of touch.

When I cared for the confused patient admitted to my unit, she slowly recognized that she was in a new and unfamiliar environment after the initial shock. She started to wander on the unit restlessly looking for the ways to leave. Her anxiety escalated to a level where she could not fall asleep during the day or night. She started to call names of people that she missed. In search for familiar faces, she entered other patients' rooms in hopes of finding someone who she knows.

In the report the next day, I learned that she continued to be restless, wandering, and constantly on the go. She slept only for ten to fifteen minutes several times during the night. She was cooperative in taking medications that so far were not effective in decreasing her anxiety. Her eyes started to look tired and I observed that the eyelids were closing intermittently when she was sitting. When she walked, her gait was unsteady and she almost lost her balance and fell on the floor. She was in a stressful cycle of agitation that could not be broken with a variety of alternative interventions.

When I looked at her in that state of restlessness, she reminded me so much of my children. The more tired they are, the more they want to move.

When they get into that cycle of restlessness it is very hard to unwind them for rest. I found that gently massaging their hands soothes them, and they are able to fall asleep in a calm, relaxed manner.

I felt that since nothing worked with this patient, it was worth trying to massage her hands. As the first step, I simply offered her my hand to hold. While she has holding my hand, I encouraged her to walk with me to her room, keeping in mind the need for a quiet environment. While she was in the room I encouraged her to lie down in her bed. To my surprise, she did. While she was in the bed, I continued to hold her hand and listened to her talk. Her thought process was disorganized but she repeatedly mentioned one name. I learned later that this was the name of her daughter who she loved dearly. While holding her hand I asked her for permission to smoothly massage her hand and she agreed. I noted that her eyes started to close and she finally fell asleep. I continued to massage her hand for the next few minutes to make sure that she went into to a deep sleep.

My heart and soul felt relieved that without more invasive interventions my patient went smoothly into a deep sleep and broke the cycle of restlessness. When I think about my children and my confused patients, I bring to my mind interventions that work for both of them. I can appreciate the importance of touch on the deeper level.

CHAPTER 42

A ROSE BY ANY OTHER NAME

BY COLEEN KENNY

"Cynthia, you're here!"

"I guess she's not having a good day, Coleen," said the concerned nursing assistant.

I reassured her that Katherine Mitchell was indeed ok. My 102-year-old friend had bestowed the nickname "Cynthia" on me based on her favorite character from the book At Home in Mitford. Cynthia was the chaplain in the story, and I considered the moniker an honor. Katherine Mitchell considered it fun when the staff thought she was confused about my name.

I met Katherine Mitchell in 2001. She was a new resident in the nursing home where I did daily rounds. She had been living with her family, but her health status now required professional monitoring. Her family visited daily and was involved in her care. The day I met her, the nursing staff had informed me that Katherine was ill. She had developed pneumonia.

Reviewing her chart, I found she had a living will indicating no heroic measures. I spoke with her family, and they were ready for comfort care. I spoke with the patient. She had a different idea. I explained to her the likely outcome of not using antibiotics. She became tearful, saying, "I don't want to die yet." Discussing the matter with Katherine and her family, we decided on a trial of oral antibiotics. This followed her wishes for no heroic or invasive measures, and also allowed a chance of recovery. She was very ill, and I began to visit daily to follow up on her condition.

Katherine slowly improved, and as her energy returned, I discovered a vibrant blue-eyed woman full of charm and wit. One of the first catch-phrases she shared with me on a day I complimented her makeup was, "Powder and paint will make you what you ain't!" I began to keep a journal of her sayings, and found myself incorporating them into my own speech.

My daily visits continued as I stole whatever moments I could to simply sit and to listen to and enjoy her. She impressed me with her knowledge of gardening, and her family brought fresh flowers from the gardens she had left behind. She also knew how to cook. I brought blueberry muffins from home, hoping to both impress her and make her feel special. Her first comment was, "Honey, how old is your baking powder?" I didn't know, but I bought a new can, and the next batch of baked goods was lighter. She was not stingy with her advice for my love life either, feeling free to question, chasten, or console depending on how things were going. She met my boyfriend, and renamed him "Father Tim" after the other main character of the *Mitford* book series. She promised to live long enough to see us married.

Katherine held an opinion on just about every subject, and she read the newspaper every day. When our state elected a new governor, her commentary was, "Money will beat brains every time!" When terrorists attacked our nation that September, she was incensed to the point I had to adjust her blood pressure and heart failure medications. I considered asking her to lay aside the news for a few days, but she had a family member very close to the Pentagon explosion, and she had the right to the news and her opinions and feelings.

Another area of interest for her was anything related to aging; she relished newspaper reports on the latest research. She had been part of a Governor's luncheon for centenarians in our state two years before, and she had also participated in a research study with a major university. Relating her contributions to an interested ear gave her joy and satisfaction.

We shared a deep Christian faith, but she was fascinated to talk to the Rabbi and learn about a different tradition in this tiny Jewish nursing home. She attended the Passover Seder that was open to all residents. She also spent time evaluating how the nursing home was run, and freely offered her advice to the administrator. She had few complaints except we could never get the coffee quite hot enough.

Katherine's birthday arrived in December. Her friends brought a cake, saying the women at the bakery made a big to-do that they had never written "Happy 103rd" on a cake before. This pleased her immensely. She was quite proud of her accomplishment.

A few months later, I received an evening call from the nursing home that I should come in. Katherine was wearing out. Her body was no longer responding to the medication adjustments I made. I was sitting by her side as she prayed. I wondered when she stopped being my patient and became my friend. She taught me so much about loving life, taking joy in each moment, having an opinion and defending it, cherishing those around you and overlooking their foibles. She personified self-determination. She reconnected my heart to nursing.

Into this quiet musing, her son-in-law and daughter entered. They greeted me warmly, telling me to stay by her side. Her son-in-law asked, "How are you doing, Katherine?"

Never removing her gaze from its heavenly bent, she replied, "Is that you, Floyd? God says hello."

Her daughter asked, "What else does God say, Mom?"

"He says there's plenty of hot coffee up there."

CHAPTER 43

AN END-OF-LIFE STORY

BY JANET M. DUDA

I will not soon forget Henrietta and Ben. The events of a morning that we spent together a decade ago remains fresh in my memory. It was one of those milestones by which we as professional nurses measure who we are, and how we feel about what we do.

The issues in long term care are somewhat different than those in acute care. It is true that there are some residents who are admitted for rehab, and it is understood that discharge planning involves returning them to their previous residences. The majority, however, are in long term care for extended periods, and in most cases, for the remainder of their lives.

The major issue of aging is loss. There is the loss of what we as humans see as important parts of living, such as health, family, and friends. Entering a long term care facility forces more loss. The majority of one's possessions are left behind, many choices of daily routine are someone else's decision, and the normal social support systems are diminished and often gradually dwindle away.

A primary focus of long term care is, therefore, to maintain as normal a life as is possible. Encouraging daily choices, retention of important personal possessions, providing activities that interest and stimulate, and participating in the maintenance of a social support system are important ways to preserve at least some of that normality.

It is the loss and social support issues that I am currently addressing.

I was the Director of Nursing of a long term care facility. Ben had been a resident at my facility for some time. He had been diagnosed with Alzheimer's disease and gradually became unable to remain at home. His wife, Henrietta, had chronic health problems and was unable to care for him. She had a son who lived locally, and who was as attentive to her as his job and family allowed. Ben was Henrietta's second husband, and he and her son had never been particularly close. Gradually Henrietta's health failed sufficiently so that she was unable to care for herself at home or to get out of the house without assistance. She agreed to be admitted to the long term care facility, although she was not happy about leaving her home, and certainly was not happy about being "put in a rest home with all these crazy people."

Normally when husband and wife are both living in long term care, we attempt to put them in the same room if they wish it. In this case Henrietta decided not to be in the same room. Ben's dementia had progressed so that he no longer recognized her consistently, and his behavior was not predictable, or even recognizable as her husband at times. So she visited as frequently as she wished.

As was my practice when new residents were admitted to the facility, I went to visit with Henrietta. I had seen her on her visits to Ben so we were not strangers, but it was important that residents knew that I was available to them for any problems. From that day Henrietta called on me frequently for all kinds of concerns, and was always happy to see me when I dropped in on my rounds. She was an unhappy, lonely woman and not always easy to deal with for some of the staff. But she and I were always able to communicate on some level and usually able to devise a solution for whatever the current problem might be.

Henrietta had been in the facility for some months when the staff reported that it looked like Ben was coming to the end of his life. He had been deteriorating slowly and was now mostly non-responsive. I went to assess his condition and had a feeling that it would not be long. Henrietta was eating breakfast in the River Room and I waited for her to finish. I approached and told her what the situation was. She seemed confused and upset and unsure what she should do. I asked her if she would like to see him and said I would take her and stay with her. She held my hand hard and said yes, she would.

I had long since noted that most of my residents, and most people for that matter, like touching and hugging any day of the week. At times of stress, physical contact becomes even more necessary.

She continued to hold my hand as I wheeled her chair down the hall to Ben's room and to his bedside. He didn't respond and his respirations were irregular. When I had Henrietta settled at the bedside and made sure she was all right, I excused myself and went out to let the staff know where I would be. I asked them to call her son and let him know what was happening, then returned to her. She was crying quietly and I sat by her. She couldn't think of anyone else to call; all of her friends were either dead, too sick to visit or, as frequently happens, had just stopped coming to visit. I thought about my normally overburdened morning schedule and made the decision that no matter what was waiting for me on my desk, it probably wasn't as important as what I was doing at that bedside.

Although death is a solitary activity and no one can do it for you, I believe that no one should die alone. People should have people with them during the really important transitions of life. If Henrietta did not wish to stay at the bedside, then I would. But she did want to stay and, furthermore, she asked if I would stay with her. Of course, I would.

For the next three hours we sat with Ben, talking, touching him, telling him that we were there. Henrietta talked about their married life. It had not always been smooth, he was not an easy man to live with. She talked about the bad times and the good times. She reminisced. She cried, she laughed, and then she cried again. I laughed and I cried along with her. I never feel bad about sharing emotions, even crying, with others whether they are patients, residents, clients, family members, or other staff, whatever the professional relationship. Never has one of them expressed regret that I did so, and almost always they express appreciation for the sharing of feelings.

After Henrietta and I had been at the bedside for about three hours, Ben's breathing slowed and finally stopped. Henrietta was calm, she had said goodbye and made her peace with him and with herself. I remained with her until her son arrived and left them quietly making the necessary plans together.

It wouldn't be the last of her tears. It isn't that easy to lose an important part of your life. She didn't magically turn into a model resident. She remained as irascible as she ever was, and there were many more problems that we had to work on. But she and I had forged a new bond, a link between us that would last until she died.

There are times and experiences that place a signature on our professional lives. In 39 years of practice I have had a few. I remember these times vividly and use them as guideposts as I encounter other lives and other situations.

This particular experience once more validated for me the importance of relationships, and the sharing of "the self" with the people to whom we give care. The therapeutic value of one heart in time with another heart during stressful moments cannot be measured. I will not soon forget Henrietta and Ben.

CHAPTER 44

MR. MONK

BY THERESA BAGENSKI

I had just secured a job in a nursing home not more than five minutes from my home. I had no idea how this job and Mr. Monk would influence me in planning my future to become a psychiatric nurse.

"Unreachable and cranky"—that was how the nurses and nursing assistants described Mr. Monk. He was small, frail looking, and angry—always angry. He sat in his wheelchair in his room day after day, leaving only to go to the front door of the facility at 6:00 am to pick up his newspaper and read it in the chapel. If the chapel was in use for whatever reason, he made an excellent effort to let people know he was not happy about this interruption in his daily routine. He ate in his room or he did not eat. He hated when visitors came to see his roommate; they never stayed long in the room because he made them so unwelcome. How lucky I was that he was on my assigned unit!

I was determined to get Mr. Monk out of his room to participate in a recreation program because there was a note on his goal chart that he should interact with others on a daily basis. I took a deep breath and started to knock on the door. It was open and I heard him say "come in." I thought, "this isn't as bad as I thought it would be." I went into his room with positive expectations and was greeted with, "What the hell do you want?" Yes, I was taken aback a little. But I swallowed hard and said I had noticed he read the paper daily and that I would like him to come down to the lounge on his floor and participate with the current events group. "No! Go away and don't come back," was his sweet reply. I quickly retreated.

Each day I walked past Mr. Monk's room, most days more than once. Usually the door was open as I passed it, I called out a "Hello!," but I kept walking, and rather quickly I might add. I do not like getting yelled at! As I would walk away down the hallway I could hear him grumbling a word or two. "Pest" was his favorite, and less colorful than most.

Each week I worked with a quilting group of five women from the same floor as Mr. Monk. I began to notice that he came into the lounge in his wheelchair. Then he scooted around the table and out of the room. After he had done this a few times, I noticed that he had been quietly taking some of the fabric squares from the boxes the ladies had been working from. I thought it curious, but thought he might be using them as hankies or for cleaning.

I was doing charts and I had Mr. Monk's chart to record his progress. I looked into his previous jobs and found he had been a handy man. Maybe this is where I need to start my work. I thought I would get him involved in the men's group with the other recreation director, Sue, and have him work with wood making toys and items for the Christmas fair. Sue personally invited him and he did go to the program, but he did not participate at all. He took the wood working kit and left the room. Sue and I looked at each other and said, "Oh well, at least he was here."

On one of our shopping trips for the department, we found an old bookcase in a flea market and thought it would be a great project for the men's group to refinish. We purchased it and brought it to the facility. But instead of giving it to the men's group, we brought it up to Mr. Monk. Sue asked him if he would help with the bookcase, as she needed it to be sanded. He told her to get out, and she did, but left the bookcase and sandpaper behind.

A few days went by and we hadn't seen Mr. Monk. We were called into the Director of Nurses office, however, and were told that Mr. Monk had been sanding his bookcase. He had left dust all over the room and housekeeping was getting upset. Rather than take the bookcase away from him, we volunteered to clean up at the end of the day for housekeeping. We also gave him a drop cloth.

Time went on and Mr. Monk was seen standing by the bookcase, sanding. He came to the recreation room more often to get more sandpaper. After two weeks of sanding, the bookcase was ready to be stained. We were so surprised when Mr. Monk came to the recreation room and helped us stain the piece.

Time went by and my husband was offered a job 200 miles away from our facility. I had to move. I said good-bye to all my residents. The facility gave a party in my honor. It was lovely and I was given gifts to remember everyone by. But the greatest gift of all was when I saw Mr. Monk wheel himself into the dining room and up to me. I had no idea what he wanted, but it soon became clear. On his lap was a quilt. I thought, 'how sweet, he made himself a lap quilt. He took it off his lap, put it on the table, and said, "Here, it is cold where you are going." I opened the quilt; it was a finished, full-sized quilt. He had made the quilt sewing it by hand. It was made with all the fabric squares that he had taken from the box of fabric that the ladies group had been working with. He was making me a quilt all the time. I felt the tears burning in my eyes. I called out to him as he left the dining room, "Thank you, Mr. Monk." He just stopped, and with out looking around, he said, "You could have stopped in when you went by saying 'hello!' " How typical of Mr. Monk to do something so nice and still stay so cranky.

CHAPTER 45

NANA

BY CATHERINE M. DUREN

Once a nurse, always a nurse! As a child I remember telling everyone that my grandmother was a nurse. My grandmother, "Nana," was a very intelligent woman and in many ways ahead of her time.

Nana was a very prim and proper lady. She always had the best stories to tell about the residents at the nursing home where she worked for many years. Nana was always working long hours and extra shifts. Often, she would work holidays for other nurses so they could spend them with their small children and families.

Years after Nana retired, she developed Alzheimer's disease and was placed into an assisted living facility. Nana was not able to stay long because she was unable to take care of herself anymore. She was then placed into a nursing home where she seemed to adapt well. I guess that with so many years working at a nursing home it was an easier transition for her than for most people, including her family.

As the disease progressed, she began living a life that may have been suppressed for many years, or perhaps was just another childhood. The once prim and proper Sunday school teacher became vivacious and young at heart again. The woman who rarely showed affection in public became a flirting school girl. She was seen chasing the maintenance man down the hall in her wheelchair. She had let me in on a secret one day. Nana had proudly told me that she and the maintenance were going to be married when they both became of age. At the previous facility, she was trying to take care of a man that she thought was my grandfather.

One of the most humorous things that Nana ever did was, one day, when the phone rang at the nurses' station and the nurse was down the hall in a patient's room giving medications. Nana scooted her wheelchair behind he station and answered the phone saying, "This is Audrey Duren, charge nurse, may I help you?" The person, or doctor, on the other end of the line began giving orders or instructions for her to carry out. Some time lapsed and the same person called back, except that this time the medication nurse answered the phone. The person asked to speak to Audrey Duren, the charge nurse. The nurse told the person that Audrey was a charge nurse at one time, but she definitely was not in charge at the present.

I am sure the entire facility got a laugh out of that and then they probably called maintenance to put a lock on the nurses' station door. Even to this day the story gets passed on by the family, and my co-workers always ask me to tell that story again. Her mind may have been deteriorating due to the disease process but she was still fulfilling her tour of duty.

The tour did not stop there. Nana had a roommate that was in a sad situation because she did not talk and was unable to do anything but lie in bed and stare. Being the dedicated and observant nurse, Nana saw that her catheter bag was filled with dark, concentrated urine. This may have indicated that her kidneys were shutting down. Nana set off to call the doctor immediately because the lady's urine didn't look right.

The other aspect that did not change was her sweet tooth—and that increased over the years. My grandparents owned and worked an old-time drug store that had a soda fountain and ice cream parlor in it. Any time that someone would go and see her at the nursing home, she would always ask for candy or cookies. The chocolate would always be found in the wrinkles around her mouth or down the front of her shirt. These are traits that I see in my father and myself. When it was time for a visit to end, she never seemed sad. She would say that she loved you and do not forget to bring her some more candy next time.

Looking back, I remember how she was always a mentor. Summer break would consist of spending a couple of weeks with her and taking walks by the old oak trees. We would go to the playground with my cousins and to the library to check out books.

One particular story I will never forget and will probably tell again and again is when we went to the second-hand store and bought some used books. The next morning, I woke up to the smell of smoke. I just knew the house was on fire. When I ran out to the kitchen I asked in a frantic way what was on fire. Nana said she tried to sterilize the books in the microwave and they caught fire. She then took them and put them into the trash and they caught fire again. That was one summer visit I will never forget. At the time, I thought sterilizing the books was the craziest thing I had ever heard. Once I became older and a nurse, the sterilization idea became clearer to me.

Looking back at all of the good times we shared together, I appreciate those moments even more. As I write this story of reflection, the tears run down my face in sadness that there will not be any more of these special moments. There are also tears of joy for the moments we did share together. Nana will always have a great place in my heart as a grandmother and as a nurse. I am also truly convinced that once you're a nurse, you're always a nurse.

CHAPTER 46

A VIEW FROM THE OTHER SIDE

BY EILEEN HESSION LABAND

"What a tough day," I said, looking for some support. "Where do you work?" she asked. "At the hospital, Mom. I'm a nurse! Don't you remember?" My mother was so proud the day I graduated from nursing school. Now she didn't even remember her daughter was a nurse.

My journey with my mother through her illness with Alzheimer's disease taught me more about nursing than I'd ever learned in school. The nurses I encountered made nursing concepts come alive in ways I had never known before: concepts like compassion, advocacy, and coordination of care. I admired nurses who anticipated and met an important and unforeseen need. I was comforted by nurses' compassionate concern. I was grateful for nurses who removed obstacles in the way of my mother's care. Witnessing these small miracles, I realized the difference that nurses make.

My journey began when my father died suddenly. Dad had been Mom's caregiver. As the nurse in the family, I felt it was my job to coordinate care and services. But after ten years in the pediatric intensive care unit, Alzheimer's was unfamiliar territory. There was so much I didn't know about home care, Medicare, Medicaid, nursing homes, and Alzheimer's itself.

My family and I faced many decisions—Who would take care of Mom? Where was the best place for her? How would we pay for it? With Dad's recent death, it seemed unwise to make drastic changes. We decided to keep Mom at home.

In addition to Alzheimer's, Mom had other medical problems. I was able to obtain a visiting nurse referral because she had a leg ulcer. Although this problem paled in comparison to her dementia, it ironically provided Medicare-funded home care. I breathed a sigh of relief knowing that Mom would have a few hours a day with a home health aide and daily visits from a registered nurse. Funding was approved for only 13 weeks. We were on borrowed time. At least the visiting nurse would help me sort through the health care maze. Or so I thought . . . .

The home care nurse seemed more concerned with changing Mom's dressings and keeping to her schedule than helping my family cope with major losses. When I asked what would happen after 13 weeks, she replied matter-of-factly, "You'll be on your own."

On our own? What would we do? Mom's modest savings would be exhausted in no time paying for home care. "You'll have to start looking at nursing homes," she said. It sounded so harsh. We weren't ready.

At my request, the nurse ordered a social services consult and we began to explore the available options. I had no idea how complex and unfriendly the health care system was until I experienced it from "the other side." I felt alone and abandoned. This home care nurse didn't live up my view of nursing. From my own practice, I knew that competence and compassion were out there somewhere.

Meanwhile, Mom had a fall and was admitted to the hospital. She deteriorated rapidly and her physician recommended nursing home placement. I didn't know where to turn.

A friend suggested joining an Alzheimer's support group. The nurse who ran it gave expert advice on selecting a nursing home, managing finances, and handling paperwork. What I found even more helpful than her practical advice was her compassionate concern. She helped me focus on Mom's strengths instead of her losses. She listened gently and nodded with understanding at my pain. She helped me to grieve when I needed to, let go when I needed to, and get busy when I needed to. I will never forget her.

Throughout our nursing home search, my heart was breaking. Putting Mom in a home? It seemed so wrong. A nurse friend noticed how upset I was one day and asked if she could help. Bursting into tears, I attempted to explain my dilemma. "If only there was another way," I said. My friend happened to know a nurse at the hospital's home care agency and put me in touch with her right away. This nurse listened carefully to my story and described exactly what it would take to bring Mom home. I wasn't sure we could do it, but I felt encouraged. She gave me a thread of hope that kept me going when reality was too painful to bear. Later on, I realized what a family I had cared for in the past meant when they said, "You gave us hope."

After several days of carefully weighing the options, we came to terms with nursing home placement as the best option for Mom. With hard work, lots of help and prayers, we found a good place for her. My first conversation with a nurse told me we were in the right spot. "What's your mother like?" she asked "What does she enjoy doing? What are her favorite foods? This information will all be included in her plan of care. And, how do you want to be involved?" She was forming a partnership with me, another way that nurses make a difference.

I often reflect on this experience and what I learned. I learned that coordination of care is more than arranging services. It's knowing the patient and family as individuals and anticipating needs they don't even know they have. It's working with them to find the best options to meet those needs.

I learned that advocacy is not just standing up for patient rights. When nurses advocate for their patients, they apply their broad-based knowledge to a specific situation. Advocacy is understanding the obstacles in a patient's way and working with the patient and family to overcome them.

Most importantly, I learned that compassion is more than kind words. It is deep concern for another person's physical and emotional well-being. It is being fully present to another in times of need. It's knowing when to offer practical advice and when to simply listen. Compassion is giving hope to patients and families and grieving with them.

The essence of nursing is all these things and more. What seems routine to a nurse seems extraordinary to a patient and family. I had never looked at things in quite this way before, but now it's clear. I know now why I chose nursing and why my mom was so proud.

Acknowledgment: The author expresses heartfelt appreciation to Judith Mitiguy, MS, RN, for being editor, mentor, and friend. Her guidance, encouragement, and thoughtful comments made this story possible.

CHAPTER 47

STUDENTS IN PROCESS

By KRISTI B. HALDEMAN

As a nurse educator of baccalaureate students, I have many wonderful experiences. One of my most anticipated experiences each year is accompanying the beginning nursing students (usually juniors in college) to the Long Term Care (LTC) facility. The students that I instruct are typically in their early twenties. Many of them have never been inside a LTC facility. Experience with elderly people is often limited among these students. As a group, the students' understanding of this arena of healthcare is minimal.

The students have spent many hours in classroom and laboratory settings preparing to care for residents in the LTC facility. They have demonstrated basic nursing skills such as bed-making, bathing, and temperature and blood pressure measurement. They are also capable of administering oral medication.

On the first day at the LTC facility, we meet in the conference room. The students' eyes are big, their expressions serious. Following an orientation to facility policies and procedures, the students must choose a resident to care for over the next several weeks. They are collectively hesitant to leave the conference room. The LTC facility staff is instrumental in guiding the students to residents who would be receptive to a student.

Jessica, a tall, blond student, chose "CeCe," an elderly woman who lived most of her life in New York. CeCe's New York accent is strong, adding to her charm. On her walls were photographs of herself from different times in her life—one of her as a young woman, accompanied by her dashing husband. Jessica frequently had to search for CeCe's dentures in the days that followed. Jessica learned the importance of dentures first hand. CeCe needed them to give her confidence in her appearance, as well as to enjoy meals and digest her meals more easily. Like many residents in many LTC facilities, CeCe easily became constipated. Jessica learned about prevention and treatment of this common ailment, but in the context of a real human being. I watched Jessica and CeCe together over the course of our LTC rotation. I observed them conversing over meals, laughing and smiling. On the days when CeCe was more subdued or not feeling well, Jessica's expression mirrored hers. Concerned and quiet, and somewhat protective, Jessica made sure CeCe's rest times were undisturbed.

Another student, Lori, was reluctantly assigned to an elderly woman who was very limited in her verbal expression. Viola often slumped over in her chair during meals. She repeated her own name again and again, the tone and volume of her recitation reflecting her mood. Lori admitted to being somewhat afraid of Viola initially. Because students are only assigned to one resident, Lori had the "luxury" of sitting with Viola for long periods of time, getting to know her and caring for her physical needs. Lori became adept at anticipating this woman's moods and schedule. Lori found that certain situations triggered Viola's more challenging behaviors. With the help of the staff, Lori sometimes prevented an agitated outburst altogether.

Viola sometimes refused one or more of her medications. Lori studied Viola, seeking a way to make medication time as smooth as possible, often with success. Although Lori began this experience tentatively, only interacting with Viola when necessary for task completion, their relationship exchanges soon had a different and deeper quality. I gradually observed the two of them, nurse-to-be and elderly woman, sitting together companionably for periods of time.

Kristin, a third student, decided to work with a frail, pleasant, 90-year-old woman named Mary. Mary's fingers were gnarled with arthritis, requiring Kristin to assist Mary with dressing and grooming. Mary's mind was quite clear. She patiently cooperated as Kristin searched to find Mary's pulse in her thin wrist, and learned to measure Mary's blood pressure. As a result of a physical assessment performed by Kristin, Mary revealed that she had great difficulty reading despite having glasses. Kristin brought this to the attention of the nurse in charge, who arranged for Mary to have an eye examination.

The students began their time at the LTC facility concerned about mastering correct skill performance, as is appropriate. They emerged with a growing competence, but, in addition, gained more than expected. Each student grew to respect and care about an elderly resident with a unique story and a unique situation, as well as unique health care needs. The students glimpsed the challenges that the staff of LTC facilities face in providing excellent care. Although this experience was one of many that they will have in their nursing careers, it was valuable and memorable—one they will never forget.

CHAPTER 48

THE FIGHTER

BY DEBRA C. WADELL

The directions on the referral seemed easy enough: 85 North to Jimmy Carter Blvd., exit and turn left. Post Apartments were on the right, approximately one half mile past Ryan's. Home health nurses are a curious breed. Good directions are an essential piece of the admission visit. Some of my favorite landmarks include churches, bridges, gas stations, and unique signs. Yes, bad directions (a turn here, a missed turn there) can cause delays and disrupt a visiting nurse's day.

The day had already had a hectic beginning. Traffic in Atlanta will give anyone a migraine and today was no exception. After our mandatory office meeting, I headed for Gwinnett County. I had called my list of patients after the meeting. (This was in 1989, pre-cell phone days!) I scurried quickly to my car and headed to my first stop of the day.

Springtime in Atlanta is truly beautiful, with the dogwood trees and peach blossoms in full bloom. As I entered Mr. Sanderson's complex, I admired the big splash of tulips. Even the small area of "greenery" in front of his apartment fashioned a lovely flower garden. Mr. Sanderson's wife, Bess, had planted the garden shortly after they had moved in.

As I knocked on the door of their apartment, I overheard a lot of grumbling and clatter. "Coming," Bess chirped. "Please, come in." I lugged in my home health bag and start-of-care packet.

Bess was a plump, slightly graying lady who appeared very pleasant. "We've been expecting you, and . . ." Her voice trailed off. She was interrupted by a gruff-sounding 60-year-old man walking toward us. "Well it's about time you got here" he glared at me as he was using his walker. Mr. Sanderson was huffing and puffing, even with the oxygen concentrator. I am always somewhat amused that patients will complain that their nurse is late, even though they are not going anywhere (they are homebound)! "My doctor said that I needed a nurse to visit me at home but I don't know why."

"Now dear," Bess explained. "You need lab work drawn, and you have a sore on your bottom."

"Oh that's right, I have a patch on my butt," he chuckled. After I did the usual mountain of paperwork, I performed a head-to-toe assessment. Mr. Sanderson was partially correct. Actually, he was sporting a crumpled gauze patch on a stage II pressure ulcer on his left hip. I measured the ulcer, cleaned it with normal saline, and applied a new patch, as ordered.

After I instructed Bess and Mr. Sanderson on the use of the oxygen equipment and the emergency planning procedure, I packed up my "tools" and informed the pair that I would return on Friday. Bess offered me a Pepsi and moon pie, a tradition that began that very day. She would offer me some type of refreshment before I left each visit. On rare occasions when my schedule permitted me linger a few extra minutes, I enjoyed eating my snack and chatting with Bess as she walked me to my car. Another ritual was Mr. Sanderson's trembling hand waving to me from his bedroom window.

I enjoyed the visits to the Sandersons. They had a supportive family. Their son James was a paraplegic, sustaining a diving injury in his early twenties. His cap collection would put Imelda Marco's shoe collection to shame! He proudly displayed them on the wall of his room. I even brought him one from New Orleans. His younger brother, Nathan, was very helpful with James's care. He even took him to Florida one summer vacation and assumed all of his physical care. Trish was the middle child. She was engaged and had an adorable daughter from a previous marriage. She would visit frequently after work.

Mr. Sanderson's respiratory and integumentary status improved and his nursing visits were decreased. One Friday afternoon around 4:00 p.m., I received a message that Bess had called the office, asking specifically for me. I was not surprised—home health emergencies always seem to occur Friday afternoons (fecal impactions that mysteriously surface before the weekend), I had practically memorized their number and quickly dialed. Bess informed me that Mr. Sanderson had seen his internist that day and was going to start insulin injections. Long-term use of steroids had taken their toll on his blood sugars. I told Bess that I happened to be on call that weekend and would be knocking on their door bright and early.

Bess had picked up all of the necessary equipment: the insulin, needles, Accucheck machine, and so on. I administered the first injection and began diabetic teaching. Bess was a swift pupil and took over the injections very shortly. Mr. Sanderson was a good soldier and was extremely compliant with his regimen.

He had truly warmed up to me over time and my visits were a big part of his life, according to his family. He refused to let other nurses visit him. Another nurse was permitted to accompany me if she were in orientation. On my colleague Glenda's first visit to the Sandersons, we discovered that they had a mutual tie—Mr. Sanderson had been in the army and Glenda's husband was a colonel in the army! Glenda's last residence was in Hawaii. This bit of information was not of interest to Mr. Sanderson, though. He was fascinated that they both had once lived in Granite City, Missouri!

It was a treat to visit Mr. Sanderson during the holidays. I was training a new weekend nurse on St. Patrick's Day and Mr. Sanderson greeted us from his wheelchair, exclaiming "top of the morning to ya!" He had a fake beard and black hat. He gave us leprechauns that he had made out of eggshells. They were truly unique! When Easter rolled around, he wore bunny ears and gave me a lavender Easter basket filled with candy!

I looked forward to my monthly visits to the Sandersons. I drew a BCP on each visit and reported the results to his physician. Those were the good 'ole days when a venipuncture was considered a "skill."

The Sandersons enjoyed hearing the progress of my first pregnancy. Their daughter loaned me all of her maternity clothes and they were gorgeous! She worked in a top-notch real estate office and her boss had given her a generous clothing allowance when she was expecting!

I checked in with the Sandersons while I was on maternity leave. He had refused another nurse to draw his blood so I performed my monthly visit! I took my baby and they enjoyed holding my two week old daughter! Approximately four weeks later, I returned to work.

That April 1st morning had been crazy. A speech therapist received a dog bite during a visit and I had to contact animal control. Another certified nursing assistant was assisting a patient to the toilet. As she was bent over, her beeper fell into the toilet.

Not realizing what had happened, the patient accidentally flushed the beeper down the toilet! I could already feel my breast milk supply dwindling as I answered the phone again.

"We're home now." It was Bess. Puzzled, I inquired where they had been. Bess informed me that Mr. Sanderon's COPD was worse and that he had to be hospitalized for three days. After work, I visited him and re-admitted him to our services. It was a sweet and sour visit. I was happy to see him but sad to see him so weak and frail. It took great effort for him to catch his breath. The disease was winning and my patient was fighting for his breath.

Mr. Sanderson died several days later. I attended his funeral service. It was nice that he was at peace, but I sure was going to miss him. He was the last home health patient that I visited regularly.

I left home health a few months later and worked at a skilled nursing facility. My former boss called me two years later, asking me to return to work. I agreed to return after I could safely leave the bathroom—I was two months pregnant with our second daughter. I visited patients when I returned but I never met anyone like Mr. Sanderson.

The gentleman who once lived in an apartment with a beautiful flower garden in the front will always remain a happy memory in my heart. From the faded Boy Scout merit badge that reads "Be Prepared" to the picture of General Schwarzkopf that was "autographed" and addressed to me, his gifts will be treasured forever. I try to abide by the Lombardi principle (it was written on a football-shaped key chain that Mr. Sanderson gave me): *Mental toughness. Control of the ball. Fatigue makes cowards of us all. Operate on Lombardi time. Make that second effort.*

Mr. Sanderson was truly #1 in my book.

CHAPTER 49

EVERY DAY

BY KAREN FONTAINE

She awoke slowly, hearing the birds—finches—fighting over the feeder next door. She kept her eyes closed, unmoving. Once she moved she knew that the pain would begin. Muscles and tissue would wake up and begin to fire their message of injury. And then it would start—the painful, dreary, unending day with only the long night to look forward to. Sleep was a fitful escape, but difficult to obtain and it evaporated quickly.

She opened her eyes and stretched to the pain pills on the table beside the chair and took two. She hadn't been able to sleep in her bed since last week. She lay back and waited for them to work. She planned her morning—the steps to the kitchen to make coffee—and wondered if she could possibly make the trip out front to get the newspapers where they had been accumulating. She also thought about what she'd do about breakfast—not that she was hungry, but she hadn't been able to drive or get to the store in a week, and the pickings were slim.

She remembered her life a month ago, the bustle of taking her friends to church and their doctor's appointments, playing bridge. She'd always had excellent health, with no real awareness of chronic pain or disability. At 85, she still had her own teeth, for goodness sake! She had kept thinking that this back pain would go away, but it got worse. Finally, she went to the doctor two weeks earlier to hear that she had broken several of her vertebra from osteoporosis. He gave her the pain pills and said there was really nothing to be done.

It was amazing and surprising to her that one person could have this much pain and still move, but she managed to sit up and get her feet under her. She got to the bathroom, and cried out as she sat down on the toilet, even though she supported herself with the sink. Getting up was easier, thank goodness. As she stood in the kitchen, she looked out at the newspapers. It was embarrassing to have newspapers lying out there, especially for her, when she was the one who always picked them up for her neighbors. She supposed that she would have to cancel—getting them from the end of the driveway was impossible now it seemed. She really couldn't concentrate anyway. The pain pills clouded her mind just enough that she couldn't follow the stories. Although she should be getting better, she felt she was getting worse and weaker. Things were getting her down, she had to admit.

She was halfway through her coffee when the phone rang. It was Gerald, her youngest son, 200 miles away. He called regularly as did her other two sons, but none of them knew about her back problem. It would only worry them, being so far away, and they had their jobs and families. She was cheerful with Gerald, listening to his troubles like she always did, and then crying a little afterward. Living alone for so many years since her husband died had created the habit of privacy, and independence. Now she was just unable to ask for help.

She was just wondering if she could manage a shower after three days without one when the doorbell rang. She thought about ignoring it, but it was her next-door neighbor, Beth, calling, "Anne? I've brought your newspapers. Are you okay?" Beth was a nurse, and did a lot of traveling. She hadn't known Beth was home, and was glad to hear her voice. She managed to get to the door and Beth looked at her for a minute and then grabbed her arm. "What's wrong?" she asked.

As Beth helped her back to the chair she'd slept in and pulled up a chair for herself, she told her everything. It was impossible not to—Beth kept asking questions that demanded answers. After she'd finished, Beth was quiet for a while and then she asked her whether she wanted her to help. Anne didn't understand how Beth could help—she was leaving again the next day on a business trip—but she didn't have any other ideas, and just hearing her story made Beth realize how desperate Anne's situation was.

Beth handed her the phone. "Call whichever son can get here the quickest and easiest. He needs to come today, or at the latest tonight, and he needs to stay until we can get something else arranged." Michael, her middle son, said he'd come that evening, after she'd explained the situation. He didn't even hesitate. She should have known he would come quickly, but got a little misty eyed with gratitude. Beth called the doctor herself and pushily made an appointment for that afternoon. "I'll go with you, and we'll see if we can get you referred for some physical therapy and a better medication." Then they talked about money. Luckily that wasn't a problem. Her retirement was adequate, and she had some money in the bank saved for emergencies. Beth said that this qualified as an emergency, and then told her she'd have to hire some help and asked if any of her friends had needed any personal help in the home. At first she said no, but on second thought, she remembered that Edina had some help when she broke her hip. They called Edina and got the name and number. Edina wanted to chat, but Beth shook her head. They needed to get her ready for the doctor.

Of course the doctor ordered the physical therapist, with Beth asking–no, insisting. Beth called the clinic to get her an appointment the next day and also to make sure that the therapist had experience working with people like her. "You mean old ladies like me," she said. "Well," said Beth, "that's the first semi-joke you've made. You must be feeling a little better."

Her son made the arrangements with the helpers. It turned out that Molly, the woman they interviewed, had several connections with people who did the same kind of work, and they arranged to be there twenty-four hours a day until she got better. They could even drive her to her appointments in her car, get groceries, and prepare meals. Michael only had to stay three days.

Beth came by to visit and check on her when she got home, and was happy at the change. She was sleeping in her own bed now, and was much more comfortable. She wasn't, however, happy with the therapist. He was "pushy," but Beth said she could handle that on her own. Anne thanked her again and again for her help, but Beth reminded her that she had done most of the work herself. "You just needed a little push."

But Anne still had one question, and she asked it. "I've been wondering if what you did for me is what nurses *do*?" "Oh, yes," said Beth. "Every day."

CHAPTER 50

THE WHITE HOUSE

BY MARGARET BONEN

So many times a person or place catches my attention, stays on the periphery of my thoughts, then lands smack dab in the middle of everything and makes me, for a time, an integral part of itself. During my nursing home care travels, I frequently drove by a white house situated on a corner lot. It had been teasing my imagination for several years. Its unkempt yard was held in by a gray metal chain link fence, like a headband reining an unruly head of fuzzy, wispy hair. A wooden ramp led to the front door, but there wasn't a gate or sidewalk leading to the ramp. I wondered if the ramp was no longer needs for my imagined old farmer. The "farmhouse" of yesterday, surrounded by the new homes of a re-zoned city, pleased my mind every time I drove past.

I received orders one morning to begin home care services for a new client. As I wrote down the address, it had a familiar ring to it, although the client's name was unfamiliar. Sure enough, the new client lived in the white farmhouse. One of the privileges of home care nursing is getting into homes you would not ordinarily be invited to visit. The instructions directed me to park in the driveway of the side street, pass through two gates and knock for entry at the enclosed back porch, and to call first so the dog could be locked up.

I followed the dirt path from the driveway around to the porch. In the corner of the path an exposed tree root had been painted bright yellow to warn against tripping. An old garden shed revealed stacks of discarded potting paraphernalia protruding through its broken windows. A dead tree dominated the side yard, left standing as a handy perch for birds after their fill at the nearby feeder. Truly this yard, with its overgrowth of plants, belonged to someone with many plans and minimal execution time.

Wooden steps lead to the glass storm door. Through the glass I could see many objects. Old wicker furniture, stacks of yellowed newspapers, last season's poinsettia plants, the old wooden screens that had been replaced years ago with aluminum storm windows, bags of water softener salt, dust, and gobs and gobs of cat hair. I knocked and waited while chastising myself for having always wanted to see the place. The porch was engulfed in cat smells. My nostrils immediately tried to forget how to smell and I promised myself it would be better inside. After all, a lot of back porches seem to gather discarded items and perhaps strays were spraying their scent on the porch foundation.

A tiny white-haired woman opened the door and she chirped a cheerful "hello." She then led me through the fur-strewn path to her sister's bedroom. My nostrils were now up to their melt-down point. The sister's room didn't change in decorating style from the porch. There were book-lined walls; junk mail lay in pyramid fashion on tables. The window sill was covered with plants and their deceased ancestors. The carpeting was patterned with cat hair. The charming old farmhouse of my imagination was dashed.

I calmed myself realizing that I was raised in a household where sweeping, washing, and airing out odors were valued. I was ill prepared to cope emotionally with this situation. In my imagination, I would trudge through a snow storm if my car failed, rather than take refuge here. I vowed never to faint during a visit so I did not accept the offer of sitting on the cat-matted chairs. Then I put my mind-shattering phobias back into their compartments, regained my nursing goals, and shut off my sense of smell. I look at the woman and feel her presence.

She is in the other world, the world of silence, the post-stroke world. This eighty-pound, 94-year-old woman, who requires total care, is living proof that cat smells don't kill. She has been in this hospital bed for ten years. Her younger sister, now in her seventies, has been her sole caretaker. Every morning the younger sister awakens to the question of whether today will be the last. She begins with a prayer that today won't be the one where she calls the funeral home. I am instantly enamored by the commitment, this basic goodness of love. There is no room for selfishness where selfless acts are the common daily rule.

I visit once a week to assess the sleeping lady's bedsores on her heels and buttocks. I carry in the needed medical supplies, advice, and emotional support. While I change the dressings, the younger sister and I talk about life, laugh about experiences, and include our sleeping beauty in all or conversations. Sometimes I can coax sleeping beauty to blink her eyelids on command. One blink is for 'no' and many are for 'yes.' This interaction electrifies us more than winning a million dollars ever could! The younger sister beams as though she has experienced the birth of her firstborn every time her sister connects with us. The sister tells me this only happens when I visit.

Sometimes, during my head-to-toe assessment, I am able to get the sweet maiden to breathe deeply for me when I listen to her lung sounds. Other times, she makes a joke and holds her breath. We all laugh, although she makes no sounds or movements, we sense her mirth.

When she takes her last breath, and I am no longer part of their life, I will neatly tuck our moments securely in that part of my being that whines about not having enough time for myself and my family. These two sisters make me know that I can have the strength and love to meet any family commitments with boundless glory.

CHAPTER 51

CRANKY LADY

BY L. M. RASMUSSEN

Think of the crabbiest, the crankiest, the most emotionally draining patient you have ever met. That was this lady. She was old. She was mean. She was uncooperative and she was (thank you) discharged from the emergency department. Finally. Had it been three hours or three days since she had rolled in by ambulance complaining of a variety of ailments that all checked out as non-existent? Yikes! I was completely wiped out by her demands and little did I know that my troubles with her had only just begun. We went round and round about who would pick her up to take her home.

Finally, after another hour of discussions she came up with a name, "Call Anne, she always helps me—which is more than you people have done!" Getting the phone number was fifteen more minutes of verbal abuse, but she did supply a number. Even though it was now 2:00 am, I called. A groggy male voice answered. I asked for Anne and he told me that Anne was not there. Not to be deterred from my mission, I boldly forged ahead. I explained that I was calling from the emergency department and we had a patient here ready for discharge who wanted Anne to help her get home. The man hesitated and then said "No problem, I'll be right in." Well, let me tell you, there were high fives all around the room. I was heralded as a genius of assertiveness.

Within ten minutes, a slightly rumpled but pleasant man entered the emergency department, stating that he was there for the patient who needed a ride. Another nurse recognized him as the husband of a long term cancer patient who had been to our hospital many times over the last year before her death. While they hugged and chatted, I went in to ready our patient for the trip home.

Her reaction was unusual to say the least. She seemed surprised that someone had actually arrived to help and asked so many questions that my suspicions were aroused. I then decided (belatedly) to double check my source and I asked her for Anne's last name. She immediately turned her head to the wall and refused to answer. Uh-oh.

After an embarrassing discussion with the nice man who came to help and a sheepish admission from my cranky patient, it turned out that she had completely made up the name and number of a caretaker. Add to that a large dose of serendipity. The fictitious number not only matched a man that had a sister name Anne, but a man who had a great respect for the hospital I was calling from and would do anything to help the nurses who helped his wife in her time of need.

After we had a good laugh all the way around (this was a *really* nice guy) he decided that since he was already up, he would still be glad to help. Our patient agreed to the plan. I'll never forget her shrill voice through the open car window as they drove away "You are driving too fast! This car is uncomfortable! Where did you get your drivers license?!" And on and on, fading in the distance as they left the parking lot.

CHAPTER 52

PEANUTS FOR JULIA

BY CLAUDIA VEPRASKAS

Julia was the only child of two highly educated Korean parents who came to the US to obtain their doctorate degrees and work. On her kindergarten registration form, her mother indicated that Julia suffered from asthma and an allergy to peanuts. No medications were ever brought to the school, however, so Julia's teacher asked me, as the one-visit-per-week school nurse, to check on this.

I telephoned Julia's father at the local university. He was a friendly and helpful man who spoke limited English. He indicated that her local pediatrician had diagnosed Julia with both conditions. Medications were prescribed and the parents purchased them some time ago. They had never been instructed in the use of either the EpiPen™ or the inhaler. Both were now expired and the prescriptions had not been refilled.

Further, they did not believe Julia really had either asthma or an allergy to peanuts. Yes, she did have a hacky cough with wheezing in the fall when severe weather changes occurred or when she exercised. Yes, she did sometimes "break out" when given foods containing peanuts. In fact, she would wheeze and cry when in the grocery store where she could simply smell peanuts. But nobody they knew in Korea had ever been told that they could not eat peanuts. Peanuts were an important part of the Korean diet. Who had ever heard of such a thing? In addition, Julia had been taken to the ER on a number of occasions due to wheezing or anaphylaxis, but they did not truly understand why these conditions had occurred. Julia, herself, did not recognize when she was getting into difficulty.

I decided that my first order of business was to convince the parents that a problem really did exist. Without their knowledge and cooperation, we did not stand a chance of implementing the necessary accommodations to allow Julia to attend school safely. Since these were educated people, I asked if they would like to receive written articles about asthma and food allergies. Julia's father agreed to read whatever I would send them. Bingo! I searched my files and got on the Internet to find several articles. I wanted to convince them but not scare them completely, so I chose the articles carefully, then put them in her backpack to arrive home that very day.

Within a week, her father called me. He agreed that the articles did "describe some of the things they saw with Julia." He expressed surprise but was now willing to listen to the recommendations. Our next order of business was to obtain current medications. He agreed to take Julia to her physician for a needed check-up and new prescriptions.

Shortly thereafter, I was presented with an EpiPen Jr.™ and a Max-Air™ inhaler by the office staff. This was my first experience with powdered inhalers, so I read up on their use, then instructed both the office staff and Julia's teachers in the symptoms to watch for and in the use of both medications. I stressed prevention as the best line of defense: use the inhaler 15 minutes prior to exercise, especially in the fall and during cold weather. Avoid projects using peanuts in the classroom (to which her teacher responded, "Oh no! We always make bird feeders in the winter by spreading pinecones with peanut butter!"). Since Julia was allergic enough that the mere smell of peanuts could trigger a reaction, we agreed that she needed to avoid sitting next to peanut-eating classmates. A plan to implement a "peanut-free table" was instituted in the cafeteria. Julia was to sit at that table every day. Anyone was welcome to sit with her, but if they carried peanuts in any form in their lunch, they ate at another table that day. The teacher's assistant monitoring lunch would be sure the table was cleaned thoroughly prior to Julia sitting down. A similar plan was adopted for snack time in the classroom.

Next, the home situation needed work. Her mother agreed to meet me at school. She cheerfully came at least four times. We reviewed physiology. We practiced with my EpiPen™ and inhaler trainers. We discussed avoidance measures. The most difficult issue was teaching her mother to use the inhaler so that she could assist Julia at home when necessary. This petite, gentle woman could only hold her own breath for two seconds. She practiced in between our sessions and eventually could proudly hold it for ten seconds. These sessions convinced me that I was not cut out to teach swimming lessons, but I was cut out to teach health and wellness.

Toward the end of the school year, I visited Julia's classroom to check on another student. It was snack time. I chuckled with the teacher as one student, in a sing-songy voice, announced, "Julia can't sit here! I'm eating peanut crackers!" Julia very willingly moved to another table without another word. It was apparent that she had learned some things herself.

It has been four years since I worked so closely with this family. They changed schools and I lost contact with them. Then, this past spring I helped another nurse with her upcoming EpiPen orders and found that Julia was in her school. I sent the required forms to her home with a friendly note to her parents. Unlike previously, I got the signed forms back almost immediately with a return note from her father. He said, "Yes, we remember you! Julia is doing so much better! She never wheezes or has trouble breathing anymore. We watch her closely during asthma season and we never have peanuts in the house."

On occasion, someone will ask me if school nurses make a difference in children's lives. Without a doubt, I believe we do.

CHAPTER 53

SWEATY PALMS

BY RUTH NELSON KNOLLMUELLER

It was early November 1961 when the arrest was made. The clinic had been open for ten days from November 1st–10th before the police entered, arrested two people, and closed the Planned Parenthood Clinic in New Haven, Connecticut for breaking the law. This began the long legal saga of Buxton and Griswold versus the State of Connecticut challenging the "blue law" that made discussion and intervention for birth control by any clinician illegal in Connecticut. The birth control pill was just completing clinical trials and not yet available, so the usual choice for preventing pregnancy was the diaphragm or the rhythm method.

I had been on the staff at the Visiting Nurse Association (VNA) of New Haven since September 1960. My typical caseload, organized around an assigned geographic area or district, was largely pre-natal, and post-partum mothers, newborns, and pre-school children, many of whom attended our Child Health Conferences for physical assessments and immunizations administered by a physician. The written policy on providing birth control information at the VNA reflected the law:

> "Any physician or nurse found disseminating birth control information or intervention would be fined not less than $50 and imprisoned for not less than 60 days, nor more than one year."

Passions on both sides of the birth control issue were verbally shrill and emotionally deep. Newspapers carried frequent releases about the plans to challenge the blue law and individuals and groups demonstrated with placards and shouts. Women, often quite young, went to the secular hospital to deliver their babies rather than the alternative Catholic hospital so that they could choose surgical tubal ligations as a way to limit the number of children they would have.

C. Lee Buxton, MD was the chief of obstetrics and gynecology at the Yale School of Medicine and the affiliated New Haven Hospital. He also was the medical director at the erstwhile New Haven Planned Parenthood Clinic. Estelle Griswold was the Executive Director for the Planned Parenthood League of Connecticut. The process in the various levels of the courts and legal system to overturn the blue law against birth control was tedious and strained. Women were asked to testify on very personal matters. Others testified against any changes in the law using the church and Bible for support. Those of us working at the VNA were informed and reminded of the limitations in our nursing practice pertaining to birth control. As nurses, we very discretely passed information among ourselves about which physicians would "help out" women asking about, wanting, and needing this information. We would mention to women that the Planned Parenthood Clinic in Port Chester, New York, a town just over the Connecticut border, was located just a block from the train station. We had to be furtive and trusting with our patients hoping none of them would report us to the police.

One especially media-focused and fervently-religious man lived on the street just next to my assigned home-visiting district with his wife and seven children. He carried placards in front of the court buildings, gave frequent interviews, and wrote letters to the editor of the local daily papers to protect the anti-birth control law. As a result, he was well known in person and in name— Mr. Miller.

One day shortly after the time of the arrest in November 1961, I returned from my day of home visiting and was heading upstairs to the office and my desk. I noticed Mr. Miller sitting near the reception desk, obviously waiting for an appointment. Halfway up the stairs I heard the secretary invite him in for his appointment to see the VNA Executive Director, Jane Keeler. My heart pounded and my palms instantly became sweaty. "Someone has reported me," I thought. When I got to my desk, I sat down, wondering how I was going to pay that $50 fine (we had been informed over and over again that the VNA would not pay it for us) and what my family would think if I had to go to jail! I would lose my job, too.

I realized I should have thought about all of that before being so helpful to those women in my district. I believed that they were sincerely asking me for guidance on family planning. I thought of Juanita, a mother of three children and pregnant with her fourth in as many years, who was desperate for help. I had visited her home just a couple of weeks before to learn that this last pregnancy caused her to "flush herself with something strong and she died in the emergency room" according to her neighbor. The impact of that experience left me shocked, angry, and feeling helpless. Now this. . . .

Some time later, I learned that Mr. Miller wanted to know the VNA policy on birth control and he was given a copy of it. No mention had been made of any breach of confidentiality from patients. Several years later I "confessed" to Jane Keeler that I had worried about what was going to happen to me and to the VNA that day. She laughed and understood what I was going through in trying to be responsive to patients by sharing information I had despite the fact that it was illegal. My angst was unnecessary, but I have never forgotten the experience.

It took until June 7, 1965 for the federal Supreme Court to rule in favor of Buxton-Griswold vs. The State of Connecticut and strike down the blue law in Connecticut making it now legal to provide all birth control services.

CHAPTER 54

PATIENT AND FAMILY VALUES

BY SANDRA MCLAUGHLIN

Recently, I had a patient who did not want to have surgery at the hospital where I worked because he would definitely need blood which was contrary to his religious beliefs. I spent the day getting to know this patient, his family, and his strong support network of friends. I got to know them as people and to understand what they held dear to them. Nobody wanted to see him die, and he certainly didn't want to die either. They just wanted the best possible care they could get. Who wouldn't!

We spent the majority of the day trying to get him admitted to the blood-less surgery hospital and requesting insurance authorization for transfer and further treatment. What a chore! Unfortunately, the insurance company did not agree that they should cover this transfer or treatment. After all, we could perform the surgery here, but no physician would touch him unless he agreed to accept a blood transfusion if required. He refused. The family waited for a final answer from the insurance company.

As I sat with this family, I was devising a plan in my head. I couldn't be the one to tell them that the insurance company was denying this transfer, if that was to be the decision. I needed to be the facilitator. I needed to be the strong one to hold everything together and to think. I needed to utilize my knowledge to navigate the system. Oh yeah, I also needed to get someone to pick up my kids. I had my husband paged to pick up my kids. My boss offered to have someone else take over. How could I do that to this family? How could I make them explain all this to someone else, and have someone else fight with them? "Thanks," I said, "but I can't do that to this family. They've been through enough. I'll be here as long as it takes."

At last, an answer. "No, we are not going to pay for that," stated the voice on the other end of the phone. I handed the phone to the wife. Again, the insurance company repeated the dreaded "No, we are not going to pay for that." What a look of exasperation on the face of the patient's wife! 'Good, I can still help,' I thought to myself. I did not look like the "bad guy." She hung up. Tears began flowing from everyone's eyes. Immediately we sprung into action; there was not a second to waste. We called the insurance company to file an expedited appeal and waited for an answer. We called the Jehovah's Witness's representative. We called the bloodless hospital to see if they would accept private pay. "No," was their answer. They wanted proof that they would get paid.

A few hours and many tears later we received a call that the decision was reversed! He could go! Now all we needed was a bed. After ten hours, we were finally on the right track!

I went home, tired and exhausted. I can't explain it, but I felt like I had given this family a death sentence originally. Mentally exhausted, I cried the whole way home and stopped a couple of times to lose what little was in my stomach. My husband asked me why I was so upset. I said, "I did not go into nursing to be a murderer. I felt like one today." He had another view. "You probably saved a life today," he said.

My patient went to the bloodless hospital a few days later. A month later I received a letter from the family saying thanks for all I did and how lucky they were to have my help.

CHAPTER 55

MILDA

By Barbara A. Stevenson

She was just 57 years old. I had gotten to know her through her multiple admissions to the ICU during my tour at Letterman Army Medical Center in San Francisco. Milda had a long history of Chronic Obstructive Pulmonary Disease (COPD) as a result of many years of smoking. Each admission was very similar—a result of exacerbation of her disease. She would be admitted in respiratory distress, be intubated, and the staff would work together to wean her off the ventilator so she could return home until the next time. But with each admission, it became harder and harder to wean Milda off the ventilator.

So it came as a total surprise to me, and the other staff members, when Milda communicated one day that her desire was to be removed from the ventilator, go home, and die. My first response was purely selfish. How could she do this to me, after all the time I had spent working with her to get her off the ventilator and get her home! Part of this reaction was related to the fact that I was still a new nurse, having been out of school just three years. I had gone into nursing to help people get well, not to help them die. The other reason I felt so upset was because I felt betrayed. After all, I had taken care of Milda for many of her admissions and wanted her to live, not to die. How could she do this to me?

Dr. Smith, our ICU Medical Coordinator, spent many hours talking to Milda about her decision. He arranged for a psychiatrist to evaluate her to make sure she was competent to make this decision. He had the social worker speak with her and her family about her decision and how she was going to be cared for after she was discharged from the hospital. He arranged for the staff, who had been working with Milda, to work with both the psychiatrist and social worker to work through their feelings and try to understand Milda's decision. After three days of consults, it was decided that Milda was competent, had made a rational decision, and was to be removed from the ventilator the next morning.

I was assigned to care for Milda the day she was taken off the ventilator. It was very hard for me and I worked even harder to make sure my disagreement with her decision was not conveyed through my non-verbal actions. Dr. Smith came in early that day and verified with Milda her decision to be taken off the ventilator. At 10:00 am, Milda was taken off the ventilator and placed on oxygen by face mask. It was hard for me to watch her struggle to breathe as I cared for her during the next ten hours. When I left at 8:00 pm, Milda was managing to breathe on her own and plans were being made to transfer her to a medical unit. It was understood by all staff members that it was Milda's wish not to be resuscitated if she stopped breathing.

When I returned the next morning I was surprised that Milda was still on the unit. I was again assigned to work with her. Also to my surprise, she seemed a little stronger. She was still on oxygen by face mask but would remove it periodically to communicate with the staff. She told me that her family had been in to see her and she knew her decision was hard on them. I took the opportunity to ask Milda why, after all the times she was admitted, weaned off the ventilator, and discharged home, did she decide to quit? Milda smiled, removed her oxygen mask and shared with me why she had made her decision. Barb, you are right, I have been here so many times and each time everyone has worked very hard to get me back home, but let me tell you what happens to me when I get home. I live by myself, my husband died several years ago, we had no children and my only family is my brothers and sister. I am close to my sister and she does come by to check on me or call me on the phone every day. I am confined to my bedroom because it wears me out walking around the house. I have a TV, which is on all the time, and now I have a commode by the bed because it wears me out just waking to the bathroom. I can't remember the last time I went out for dinner, or to shop, or go to a movie. I have the time but just don't have the energy or money to do anything else but exist. I have finally decided that I do not have a "quality" life anymore, so I just want to live out my life, be comfortable, and let God take me whenever he is ready."

"Quality of life"—That term stayed with me throughout the remainder of the day. As I drove home, I finally realized, and could accept, the reason for Milda's decision. I suddenly felt guilty for putting my feelings ahead of Milda's. I decided right then and there to do whatever I could to help Milda get home.

The following day, as I again cared for Milda, I thanked her for sharing with me the rationale behind her decision. I also promised to help her in any way I could to get her out of ICU, up to the medical unit, and home. I realized that it was much easier to care for someone if you have the same goals. I was also an advocate for Milda with the other staff members, helping them to understand her decision. Milda stayed in the ICU for two more days. The last day I took care of her she wanted me to celebrate her discharge when the time came. I promised her that I would. She told me that she would call me the night before she left the hospital and wanted me to come and share a meal and a glass of wine with her before she went home. In the time we had spent together we discovered our love for the wines of California. I told her, "just call me and I'd be honored to share a glass of wine with you."

One week later, I received a call from one of the nurses on the medical unit. She had a message for me from Milda. Milda was being discharged the next day and she wanted to remind me of the promise I had made to her before she left the ICU. She asked if I would be able to come have dinner (yes and wine) with her that evening. I told the nurse I had to work until 7:00 pm but could come up after my shift was over if that was okay with Milda. The nurse called me back and I had a 7:30 pm dinner date with Milda.

I don't remember what we had for dinner. I do remember the wine, though. It was a Merlot, Milda's favorite. She had asked her doctor for an order to drink a glass of wine with dinner before she went home. She had her sister bring the bottle of wine from home. During the meal, we laughed, cried, and talked about her going home. I felt she was at peace with her decision and was ready for whatever was going to happen. The doctor and nurses had promised to keep her comfortable because she was afraid she would be in a lot of pain. I thanked her once again for being my teacher and for helping me to realize that my role as a nurse is more than helping people get well, it is also helping them die with dignity and comfort.

Milda was discharged the next day. I called her one time after discharge and she told me she was getting along fine "in my room." Milda passed away approximately two weeks after discharge. I was sad but happy for Milda and thankful our paths had crossed.

It was thirty years ago that Milda and I shared that glass of wine. Now as a school of nursing faculty in a baccalaureate nursing program I share Milda's story with my students, especially when we talk about death and dying. But Milda's lesson has not only helped me in teaching my students, it helped me when my own father passed away by allowing me to help my family understand "quality of life."

Thank you Milda. I'll never forget you.

CHAPTER 56

DISCHARGE PLANNING

BY ELLEN R. THOMPSON

A patient's medical insurance benefits often dictate the type of arrangements a hospital discharge planner is able to make. Because of this, discharge planning can be challenging and frustrating. Bob's story illustrates the complex dilemmas faced by discharge planners and hospital patients in today's health care delivery system.

Bob was admitted post-operatively to the hospital surgical floor after undergoing an urgent esophagectomy for throat cancer. A tube was placed into his stomach at the time of surgery. I was Bob's discharge planner and my job was to ensure that all patients had discharge plans arranged by the time they were medically stable for hospital discharge.

Bob's medical insurance benefits covered his surgery and hospital postoperative care. After discharge, however, his insurance didn't cover Bob's tube feeding nutrition, which he might very well need for the rest of his life. Bob's surgeon expected me to find a way for Bob to afford his artificial nutrition despite having no insurance coverage for it.

Bob was in his mid-thirties, single, and lived alone in a mobile home. He had no family in town, and didn't want to ask for help from his out-of-town family. He worked full-time as a merchandise stocker for a national retail store. Bob had managed his life, thus far, independently.

The long-term consequences of Bob's illness were difficult for him to grasp. He was slated for a hospital stay of five days. His first and second days were spent beginning to walk, managing pain, assessing his respiratory status, and encouraging hydration, while waiting for bowel function to return. Tube feeding began on the third day after the surgery with a diluted formula. The formula was quickly increased in both rate and concentration because Bob tolerated it well. He was medically and surgically ready for discharge on his fifth post operative day.

Bob had several significant barriers to discharge. Foremost, communication was a huge barrier to planning Bob's discharge. His voice gradually improved and was somewhat understandable by the fourth day with a lot of effort. At discharge, he was still unable to talk over the phone. In his first three post-op days, Bob's perspective about discharge almost entirely consisted of wishful denial of any need for assistance that was demonstrated by his lack of interest and his rare eye contact during my visits. But as he watched the nurses begin to hang his nutrition, and adjust his feeding pump, and as he began to talk to the nutritionist, he came to slowly accept the idea of getting help after his discharge. Because he couldn't talk very much or very clearly, it was difficult to assess his level of understanding and his ability to cope. He seemed able to listen to information about his feedings and the care of his wound, but his responses continued to show an element of denial. For example, on the fourth day Bob said, "I won't need nurses at home. The doctor says the tube feedings are easy to do."

Bob's lack of a support system was another discharge problem. He qualified for a few home care nurse visits to assess his nutrition, his hydration, and his wound. The home care nursing plan also continued education about tube feedings. John's medical insurance would not authorize home nursing visits beyond the first two weeks at home because his wound could then be monitored at the surgeon's office on a weekly basis. Once Bob could drive, he wouldn't be homebound any longer, and his benefits didn't include support for tube feedings.

Bob's only other support system was the surgeon's office. The surgeon's office nurse, Linda, ended up making a home visit, which helped decrease Bob's sense of being alone to sort out a complicated medical situation. She was willing to talk to Bob on the phone, and helped him when he came to their office with questions or problems. This situation was a catch-22 for Bob. Talking on the phone was very frustrating for him, because we couldn't understand him very well and often had to guess what he was trying to tell us. Yet, a visit to the hospital or to the surgeon's office for anything except an official doctor visit broke his homebound status and terminated his homecare support.

Bob's third discharge problem was not having benefits for tube feedings after hospital discharge. His medical insurance policy stated that tube feedings were equivalent to normal nutrition and since the insurance company didn't pay for normal groceries, they wouldn't cover Bob's tube feedings. By Bob's fourth hospital day, I had talked to the nutritionist, the nurses, and the surgeon, apprising them of Bob's lack of coverage for nutritional needs.

Another discharge challenge was that Bob would be unemployed for several months recovering from his surgery and radiation. His inability to talk clearly, and altered facial appearance were also a potential barrier to rapid return to employment. Bob's expenses of rent, utilities, car payment, and all the other mundane costs of daily living wouldn't stop, but his income had.

In order to facilitate a smooth, non-traumatic transition to his home I asked the nurses and nutritionist to change his formula to a more inexpensive brand, and also to change his feeding style to an intermittent system in place of a continuous drip, so he would not need a feeding pump. Both of these changes had the potential to delay Bob's discharge, because any change in formula and any change in volume required an adjustment in Bob's bowel absorption and could have caused Bob to have diarrhea. Fortunately, they didn't. Once Bob began on bolus feedings, his nurses began to teach him how to administer the formula, how to check for residual formula, how to clean his equipment for repeat use at home, how to follow his formula with water, how to crush his medications so they would fit through the feeding tube, and how to care for his healing stomach wound. Understandably, all of this education was almost overwhelming for Bob as he anticipated going home alone. He mastered the feedings, the water administration, and the medication crushing and mixing. He was a little more careless on equipment cleaning and reuse. He had difficulty recognizing the symptoms of wound inflammation, cleaning it, and keeping track of his hydration via his urine and stool composition.

While Bob was still in the hospital, I asked his insurance company's on-site RN case manager to request an exception in Bob's situation, to ensure that he would have access to adequate nutrition after discharge. Bob's surgeon wrote a letter, which I gave to the RN, documenting Bob's continued medical need for tube feeding nutrition as 100% of his calorie and fluid intake. In theory, coverage of Bob's formula would benefit the insurance company by improving Bob's recovery time and decreasing his risk for complications that will occur if a patient with wound healing has poor nutrition. By the time of his discharge, this request had not received a response.

Bob went home with a patchwork of temporary plans for his care. His discharge pain medication had to be specially approved for insurance coverage since the liquid tube feeding form of the medicine was not on the insurance company's standard plan but Bob couldn't swallow standard pills. The hospital nurse discharged him late in the day so that he would not need a homecare nurse visit until the next morning for his tube feeding administration. The hospital sent home a one-day supply of formula for Bob. The hospital also approved an arrangement with a medical supply store to supply Bob's ongoing need for formula and bill the hospital for an indefinite period of time. Hospital administration approved this request after Bob completed a financial worksheet that documented his lack of resources and income. Bob's surgeon's office also donated almost a full case of formula that another patient hadn't used. With these unique, temporary arrangements, Bob was discharged.

I followed Bob after discharge for several reasons, none of which are in the standard discharge planner job description. Since I initiated and justified the plan for the hospital to pay for Bob's enteral nutrition, I felt responsible to make sure that Bob was successful in using this arrangement. Bob did have some initial confusion about how to tell the store's retail clerk to bill the hospital for his formula, because not all of the clerks were aware of this very unusual arrangement. Bob's voice was still difficult to understand, and he was uncertain about how to explain the details himself. After the on-site nurse case manager told me that her supervisor had denied the request for an exception for benefits, I asked her if I could contact Bob's insurance company directly. She took my request for this information back to her supervisor and returned in a few days with several suggestions about how to make the contact.

The first idea was to call the local store of Bob's employer and talk to his manager. His manager was on vacation when I first called. I left a voice mail and followed that up a week later with another phone call. Bob's manager responded to my description of the situation with interest and empathy, but he was unsure how and with whom to communicate Bob's lack of benefits for medical needs. He told me that he would contact me after talking it over with the regional store's human resources department in a different city. I contacted the local store manager again the next week. He told me he hadn't gotten any answers yet. He assured me he would leave another message with his human resources department. Next, I received a call from the district human resources representative assuring me they would check into Bob's situation and assist him in all possible ways. He seemed to be telling me that I didn't need to concern myself about Bob any further.

At this point I gladly put my concerns about Bob's nutrition at the back of my mind. My job was always to focus on inpatients' needs, and to assume that at discharge, someone else or the patient themselves could be capable advocates. As time passed, however, my department continued to receive bills for the tube feeding formula, and Bob maintained contact with me so that I still occasionally wondered about what had occurred after I had talked to his human resources representative.

After several months, my curiosity motivated me to locate Bob's medical records file and look through my notes for the phone number to his company's human resources department. I called them and learned that my appeal to give Bob coverage for his tube-feeding nutrition had not been followed. The human resources person told me that she would contact the nurse case management department within the store's hierarchy and ask them to contact me. And finally, eureka! Talking to the nurse was like balm to my sense of fatigue about Bob. She said she was sorry I hadn't been initially directed to her department, which was where situations like Bob's were reviewed and acted upon. With the surgeon's letter documenting Bob's need for tube feeding and the knowledge that cancer had caused this need, Bob's employer gave him the benefit exception and made it retroactive. All the bills that my hospital department had paid were reimbursed. Bob's company's case management nurse made an arrangement with the medical supply store from which Bob was getting his formula. The store was to bill Bob's employer directly.

I was happy and relieved that at last I could put Bob's concerns aside and attend fully to my current patient load. My discharge planning responsibilities had been completed and Bob had access to his nutrition for as long as he would need it.

For many nurses, a relationship with a patient doesn't automatically terminate at hospital discharge, especially if the patient is at risk of failure without a nurse's continued advocacy. Defining boundaries is one of the most difficult challenges for nurses. This is a personal and professional gray area. We often find fulfillment and professional rewards in helping our patients. But advocacy consumes time and energy, and after not receiving responses to my appeals, I often second-guessed my course of action. I am glad I persisted because not only were my efforts successful, but I felt more optimistic that one person really can make a difference.

Several months later, I received a letter from Bob's medical insurance administration. They thanked me for my appeals for tube feeding formula coverage for Bob. Because of these appeals, his employer changed their health insurance policy to cover nutritional formulas and supplements nationwide for the diagnosis of cancer. I had never considered that my individual efforts might influence anything more than Bob's individual case. I was reminded again how rewarding the nursing career can be.

CHAPTER 57

PASSOVER AT THE COUNTY JAIL

BY MARLA GUNDLE

Every morning at the large urban county jail where I work as a nurse practitioner, we see ten to twenty inmates who are undergoing severe alcohol withdrawal. Suddenly stopping alcohol use when arrested can lead to a great deal of physical discomfort, seizures, even death, but medication, fluids, and frequent skilled monitoring can decrease the dangers.

Usually it takes many years of hard drinking before someone has a really terrible withdrawal from alcohol, but occasionally a younger person with the "right" genes and enough of an alcohol history will also have a bad time when consumption ceases. A few days before Passover, I was assigned to work in the infirmary where I took care of Dave, a young man in his late 20s. The patient was having such severe withdrawal symptoms that he was not able to go to the clinic to be seen by a physician, the usual procedure.

As I spoke with Dave about how I could help him with his nausea, diarrhea, and tremors, I sensed there was something he was trying to muster up the nerve to ask. As we talked, we discovered that we were both Jewish. He blurted out a concern about getting access to matzah for Passover during his incarceration. We spoke a bit about the Seders of our past as I pondered what to do.

With his permission, I placed a call to the rabbinic chaplain on call. The Rabbi was extremely harried with pre-Passover stress in his voice. He was very clear that he simply would not drop some matzah off at the jail for Dave until he was sure that Dave was really Jewish. It seems inmates of other faiths try to get kosher food, thinking it might be of a higher quality.

I handed the phone to Dave, who through his tremors and nausea, began to recite, on the Rabbi's request, the names of his mother, father, grandparents, the date of his Bar Mitzvah and other pertinent facts. The Rabbi was not completely satisfied and wanted to call Dave's father. Dave became agitated. His eyes caught mine and he pleaded, "No! It will kill him if he knows I'm here — he's got a bad heart." He began to cry and handed the phone back to me, tearfully saying that all he wanted was a single piece of matzah. By now, regretful to have initiated this process, I also understood that Dave was terrified his father would find out about his legal problems and the alcohol use that caused them.

The determined Rabbi wanted to try again, so Dave spoke with him. At the Rabbi's request he began reciting Hebrew blessings, ones learned for his bar mitzvah at age 13. There in his soiled jail garb he bobbed back and forth, shifting uncomfortably until the Rabbi was satisfied that Dave was Jewish. When Dave hung up, we both looked at each other in amazement. I wished him "Chag Sameach" (happy holiday) and a speedy release from jail.

Dave enjoyed his matzah. His parents probably still don't know he drinks too much.

CHAPTER 58

I GET UP SEVEN TIMES

BY EVA OI WAH CHAN

I first met Jane at a community center. I was invited to the center to deliver a talk on mental illness to a group of volunteers who would offer services to mental patients at the hospital. The program coordinator told me that she had arranged two sessions for that evening. The first session was my talk on mental illness. The second session would be conducted by a patient who would share her personal experience with the participants. I was invited to join that session as well.

The group of volunteers and I moved from a classroom setting to a sitting room following my talk. All participants were excited to meet this second speaker, as it probably was the first time for them to chat with a mental patient in such an informal setting. After waiting for about 15 minutes, a Chinese lady walked in the room with the program coordinator. She was introduced to the group, and said, "My name is Jane."

Jane was middle-aged. She was small in build and dressed in casual wear. She was so slim that, at first glance, I guessed she might be suffering from anorexia nervosa. She had set her hair in a traditional style and appeared slightly old fashioned. She spoke in a soft voice and sounded a bit anxious at the beginning of the conversation. She started to introduce herself and recounted the history of her illness. She talked spontaneously and gradually began to smile from time to time. She became more relaxed when she shared her homemade snacks with us. She told us, "I like cooking very much. I had attended various cooking classes at this center and won some awards for my cooking."

Yes, it was true. I believed that she had very good cooking skills and her snacks were delicious. While we were eating the snacks, we were motivated to listen to her story. Everyone in the room could feel her friendliness and was ready to be her listener.

Jane actually had suffered from schizophrenia for more than 20 years. She worked as a manager at a financial company when she was young. She was bright and highly competent in her work. However, it was very stressful to handle all the issues in the commercial market. She had married and had a baby boy at the onset of her illness. Her work performance gradually deteriorated when she had insomnia. She felt that she was being blamed by everyone at the office without any appropriate reason. She even ended her relationship with relatives or had quarrels with them repeatedly.

She was so exhausted that some negative symptoms began. She had little motivation or energy at that moment for her daily life. Her mood turned to its lowest level. She was severely depressed at that moment, and thus, she attempted suicide seven times. She remembers that she jumped from an overpass at her last attempt. She was badly injured but her life was saved.

She had stayed at the hospital for treatment and rehabilitation for several months after that horrible attempt. She could not move. She had to be in bed 24 hours a day. It gave her plenty of time to stare at the ceiling and think about her mental illness. She started to review the different phases of her life. There was happiness and sadness. No matter how much pain she felt from her injuries, she still felt a lot of warm helping hands from her family members and hospital staff.

She recalled, "The nurses had spent a lot of time with me. They looked after all my activities of daily living, from morning toilet to bedtime bath; from breakfast to night meal; from oral medication to physical exercises. In addition, they did not just care for my body but for my mind as well. They gave reassurance and encouragement to me from time to time. They gave me nonverbal messages that I was special when they carried out different bedside tasks. I don't know how to describe the message, it was just something that I could feel from their touch."

Jane continued to share what made her change her attitude toward life. "I was down one night. I was preoccupied with all the unhappy events in my past and cried. I couldn't dry my face because my arms were in casts. A nurse came to change my position, and found me so upset. She then sat by my side and sang some hymns to me."

"I have forgotten the name of that hymn, but, I always remember its content. It says that God would forgive us seven times and seven times. As you know, I have attempted suicide seven times and I am still alive. I really think that God has given many chances for me to rebuild myself. I decided to cheer up. I don't want God doing extra work for me any more."

"Besides, the nurse sang another hymn for me:

In this world of confusion, discontent, disillusion,
do you have what it takes to be free?
There's a life that's worth living. There's a way of forgiving.
Just let Christ be your Master; then you'll find what you're after
and you'll have what it takes to be free.

The nurse had a very sweet voice and my distress was relieved as she was with me for about 30 minutes. I felt very touched that night. Although the nurse had not given any medication to me, it seemed that some strength had been injected into my body and mind. I started to perceive that there could still be hope in my life."

Jane made many changes after that hospitalization. She took some courses at the community center. She became aware of her skill and interests in cooking. Her confidence increased as she won various awards in cooking competitions.

She emphasized, "I was happy to get all those awards not because of the prizes, but because they helped me to redefine my personal value. Credit had to be given to my family, too. They had encouraged me to participate in different activities. My potential was fully developed under their continuous support."

Jane and I have kept in contact occasionally since then. We became closer when we worked together on some social activities for mental patients from time to time. Now Jane is an active member of different voluntary organizations that promote mental health and give positive messages to the public. She has been interviewed by newspapers and radio shows, sharing her experiences. She encourages patients and clinicians in the field of mental health services. It is important to maintain hope for our patients even in the face of a long history of illness.

CHAPTER 59

THE DEVIL'S EXCOMMUNICATION

BY KATHY WILMERING

The sterile environment of the 2-South county psychiatric unit receives patients who are involuntarily hospitalized with mental health disorders. People are placed there against their will but only when, as a result of a mental illness, their behavior directly threatens their safety or someone else's. Most people with schizophrenia, bipolar disorder, and other chronic mental illnesses do no harm to the public, and if they harm anyone, it is usually themselves. Only a small percentage of these patients harm others; many studies conclude that except for paranoid schizophrenia, people with mental illness are no more likely than the general population to harm someone. Still, persistent severe mental illness saps a person's finances and relationships; patients admitted here are disproportionately poor, homeless, and alone.

The journey begins as the patients arrive in the emergency room, rousted out of their environment by the police or anxious relatives. Some arrive mute and unreactive; others curse, scream, bite, spit, hit, and throw whatever objects are at hand. A few relax in clear relief, free of bearing the heavy burden of keeping themselves and others safe from their uncontrollable impulses. Sequestered in a locked, sparsely furnished room, they may be placed in leather restraints if no other intervention contains them. We do what we can to calm them: talking gently or firmly as the situation requires, discovering what friend or relative they'd like us to call, keeping the environment as low-key as a part of the ER can be.

A 2-South RN staff member arrives to transfer them. The shame of their restraints covered by a sheet, they are presently wheeled through the ponderous double doors of the unit, which thud shut and lock directly behind. The journey ends in a barren locked room, sparsely furnished so that they have no items with which to hurt themselves or others. Stimulation is kept to a minimum. The staff joins together to transfer the person to his or her bed as safely as possible. Getting assaulted by confused or angry patients is a routine risk of the job.

We make the person as comfortable as possible and check on them every 15 minutes. We do a thorough physical and psychosocial assessment that includes a list of the patient's strengths and family resources, though sometimes neither is obvious upon admission, and when possible, notify relatives that the person has been admitted.

One woman in her late fifties had no family. Her matted hair and parched lips in her worn face eloquently conveyed the tale of her long struggle with chronic schizophrenia. Often tormented by voices and visions that foretold great harm to her, she had tried to destroy them by setting her apartment on fire.

From the time of her admission to the ER she had screamed and screamed. My imagination puzzled over how she avoided losing her voice. "The Devil! The Devil!" she would shout in great panic, screaming that he was here and was already hurting her. Alternately curling up and lashing out, she screamed through the night. When I came in again on Sunday morning, the night staff reported that despite massive amounts of antipsychotics (medications used to stop hallucinations) and sedating drugs, she still had not slept or slowed down. All the reassurances of each staff member had done nothing to calm her. No distraction seemed to soothe, and she couldn't tell us if she had any spiritual beliefs that we could help her mobilize.

On a busy weekend when weary staff have unsuccessfully tried every intervention they can think of, it is tempting to stop efforts to comfort patients as the screaming becomes a routine part of the background. I went in to check on her and felt a surge of helpless compassion for her intense suffering. "The Devil!" she sobbed loudly, pointing to a spot toward the window.

An idea popped into my head. I straightened my back to its most rigidly regal stance and in my best haughty, authoritarian voice announced, "The Devil is not approved for visitation on 2-South. He will not, under any circumstances, be allowed on the unit." "But—he's right here!" she sobbed frantically. "No. He always tries to pull that. He's actually out there." I pointed beyond the chain-linked windows. "He'd like to think he can get in here, and he always tries to make people think he has." "No, he's here," she screamed hoarsely. "Do you remember those enormous double doors you went through to get in here?" I asked. "Yes." For the first time her screaming paused a bit. "And how they made that big bang and locked behind you?" "Oh, yes," she shuddered. "Well, those doors have been specifically Devil-proofed with new patented technology. He's tried for years to get in here, but since we installed those doors, he has found it impossible. And he is not on the approved visitors list, so he can't get in that way either." She was completely silent, her eyes big as she stared at me in surprise. "So each time he tries to fool you into being scared, you just tell him what you know." This time she accepted a drink of water and stayed calm the rest of the shift. By the time I worked my next weekend, she had been transferred and no one remembered where she had gone.

CHAPTER 60

JUST CALL ME SARAH

BY PAMELA STURTEVANT

This morning, in the light of a butter-colored sunrise, I found a blue jay feather, lying like a gift on a patch of wooly thyme. I picked it up and held it to the sky. Tickling my chin with it, I felt the dainty whisper of forgotten things. In those cerebral flutterings, I remembered Marie.

Marie was my patient years ago, when I worked on a cardiac unit of a local hospital. She had heart disease and Alzheimer's and was admitted to us from a nursing home because of fainting spells. Her heart stumbled along in an irregular rhythm, causing the cardiac monitor to ring frequently.

Past memories and confusion obscured her mental state. She fidgeted from the restless energy of dementia. When I arrived for the 3 pm to 11 pm shift, she was sitting and secured in a chair in the hall, across from the nurses' station.

"Timmy! Timmy! Where are you?" cried Marie. Physicians passed her with straight-ahead faces and sideways eyes, wary of contact. Visitors gawked as though she were on display. "Timmy! Have you seen Timmy?" she beseeched to everyone and to no one. She received a few mumbled responses of "No, I haven't seen him."

As soon as I finished report, I headed straight to Marie to check her vital signs, give medication, and assess her mental status. While she was engaged with me, she momentarily stopped calling out. I didn't mention Timmy, hoping it was a passing agitation.

As I continued on my rounds, she remained quiet, but active in her quest to get out of the chair. She leaned over its arms, looking underneath the table that trapped her, and asked a passing person for a screwdriver. She pulled and tugged at her vest restraint calling out for scissors. She had escape plans.

Then "TIMMY! TIIIMMMMYYYY!"

The nurses at the far end of the hall, on the respiratory unit, poked their heads around the corner of their nurses' station. Visitors stood in doorways. My colleagues looked at me with sympathy and a palpable relief at not being in my shoes. I had four other patients in various stages of cardiac disease plus Marie.

Supper trays arrived at 4:30 pm I checked my other patients to make sure everyone was set up and eating, then settled down next to Marie. Although she was physically capable of feeding herself, food had no meaning to her anymore. She played with her napkin instead. I asked her who Timmy was. "Oh Sarah, you know Timmy—my little cat. He's outside and it's so dark. I'm worried about him," she said.

Gently correcting her, I said, "Marie, my name's Pamela, not Sarah." She looked at me vaguely, her blue eyes faded and distant as she struggled to process this information. Her agitated fingers tore the napkin into bits of white snow. She started squirming and tried to stand up. I decided to be Sarah for the rest of the shift, if that would calm her.

"Marie," I said, "I'm going to look for Timmy while you finish your dinner." Her look of gratitude was heart wrenching.

"Oh, thank you Sarah," she cried. "Check the back porch!"

I wandered down the hall, peering behind laundry carts. I opened closet doors and stuck my head into the kitchenette. "Timmy, Timmy, here kitty," I called softly. I glanced back at her and noted she was fixed on my progress with great concentration. Her dinner was untouched. I ducked into the patient lounge and waited for a couple of minutes.

When I returned to the hall, she was quiet and focused on the lounge doorway. I strode confidently back to her. "I found him, Marie, He's safe and you were right, he was on the back porch. I gave him his supper and now he's curled up on the couch, on that little blanket he likes"

"He likes it there, doesn't he, Sarah," she said with a broad smile. "And he's alright?"

"Yes, he's fine," I said taking her hand. "I checked him all over—not a scratch."

"Is Joe with him?" she asked.

"Yes, he's on the couch too, watching television, while Timmy sleeps." The story was becoming easy now.

"Oh, I'm so glad he's there with him." Her lips folded in and out of her toothless mouth. She ate her meal with a little prodding, and then sat quietly sipping a cup of tea and moving napkin pieces around her table, as though concentrating on a game.

The evening continued in relative calm. No miracle happened to change Marie's condition. She went in and out of restless phases, but never called out again for Timmy. She would ask about him sporadically, seeming reassured by my answers.

When I finally sat down to write my notes, I tucked her chair next to me and bundled her in blanket shawls and lap covers. She ate vanilla ice cream with child-like enjoyment, and then folded a small pile of clean facecloths into perfect squares, her hands ironing with repetition.

I finished my notes at 10:30 pm and turned to her with a tired smile and little wink. Still awake and watchful, she asked if I had finished my homework. Laughing I told her that, yes, it was finished at last. She reached out a trembling hand, finger joints swollen and twisted with arthritis, and softly, with the barest hint of contact, caressed the skin under my chin. I thought of feathers and summer breezes.

"I love you, Sarah," she said. "You look tired. Why don't you go lay down on the couch."

I helped Marie to bed, tucked her in, and told her that I would sit on the couch for a while with Timmy and Joe. Her eyes sparkled in the night light as she took my hand and held it against her cheek. "Good night, Sarah." "Good night, Marie."

I placed the feather back on the pillow of thyme and watched the sky turn a golden color and heard the birds call. The same quiet joy filled me, as it did those years ago, when I entered Marie's past, easing her anxiety with reconnection to her long-dead husband and her cherished pet. If there are guardian angels somewhere in this great life, I will feel truly blessed if mine is a gentle lady who calls me Sarah, and carries in her beautiful, withered hands, a little cat.

CHAPTER 61

PRISON STRESS MANAGEMENT

BY IRENE O'DAY

When I retired from nursing ten years ago, I looked forward to a well-deserved rest. My dear friend and spiritual director, Sister Pat had other plans. She invited me to join her as a volunteer in her ministry at the state prisons where she serves as chaplain. Since all of my talents involved nursing, I wasn't sure what I had to offer. I had kept up with holistic nursing and could do therapeutic touch, visualization, guided imagery, and music for healing. With Sr. Pat's encouragement, I was able to introduce some of these modalities during days of reflection at the women's prison, and more recently at the men's prison.

Two years ago, Sr. Pat asked me to develop a program for the men using meditation for stress management. Because some of the men have a history of heavy drug use, short attention span, limited education, or a language barrier, I was asked to keep instructions simple, clear, and concise. These are never obstacles for a nurse; so I created a program.

The program is called "Meditation for Stress Management" and includes breathing exercises, progressive relaxation, visualization, guided imagery, music, prayer, and silent meditation. We meet in the prison chapel for one and one-half hours each week for eight weeks. The program is limited to 25 men and there is a waiting list. Each man is given a certificate of completion that is placed in his record.

I use a neurophysiologic approach, rather than a psycho-spiritual one, as I know little about the latter. I begin with a simple definition of stress and its effects on the body, mind, and spirit. Pictures, diagrams, and handouts help explain the concepts. Thanks to my husband and engineer son, I learned a few military and mechanical terms. I already had some prison jargon and was able to explain the medical aspects of the lessons quite effectively. I was amazed at how quickly the prisoners grasped the concepts and began using words like immune system, endorphins, and hypothalamus. One man surprised me with a poster of the brain with all parts labeled and colored. He had created it in another class with his teacher's assistance.

Because I wanted to introduce the Mozart Effect, I wondered how classical music would be received. Thanks to a synchronistic connection at my public library, I discovered a Mozart CD with the music featured during a high point in the movie, "The Shawshank Redemption," a brutal prison movie. Most of the men had seen the movie, which is shown often. I played the piece, "The Letter Duet" from the opera "The Marriage of Figaro." I asked them to close their eyes and imagine the music flowing through their compound, as it did in the movie scene. They listened with contented faces, some smiling. When the music ended, they related visualizing scenes of peace, cooperation, and good will in an area usually full of tension and stress. One man volunteered to read the lines from that scene in the movie, which were printed on the CD jacket. That added a dramatic note to the experience. They tell me now that when the movie is shown, they look forward to that scene.

As the sessions progressed, the shared experiences were deeply moving. Before incarceration, Russ was an IV drug user who could inject himself, but could not tolerate any invasive attempt by any one else. Twice he was scheduled for excision of two suspicious skin growths, but panicked before the procedure was started. Threatened with loosing his privileges, he tried again, using the techniques he learned in our program. To the amazement of the medical staff, he calmly underwent the excisions. Afterward, he suggested the staff attend our sessions.

Dave suffered from severe, chronic constipation, partly due to poor diet and the lack of privacy in the group toilet area. I counseled on diet changes, increasing fluids, and suggested specific visualization, along with relaxation techniques. At the end of the program, he excitedly announced that his problem was much improved and received a round of applause.

The men are always courteous, respectful, and expressed deep gratitude. I feel safe and protected at all times. There is a special reverence in the chapel where we meet and at times we experience moments that are profound and luminous. After each session, I am left with a feeling of awe and a deep sense of purpose. Every nurse experiences brief moments of transcendence while caring for patients. I am blessed to have the opportunity to serve in this way. The greatest gift these men give me is the feeling that I used to have on the best days of my nursing career.

CHAPTER 62

KNOWLEDGE IS POWER

BY PEGGY S. CAMPBELL

I have a sister who is deaf. Knowing sign language has been very helpful in my life and my career. When I was in nursing school, during the first week of psychiatric rotation, we were assigned to the men's ward. As students, we gathered at the nurse's station every morning to listen to report. Shift report occurred three times daily. The shift going off duty gave a report on the patients to the shift coming on duty. I took notes during shift report, spent time reading patient medical records, and got acclimated to the ward.

After a few days I became more comfortable with the environment and was able to spend more time observing what was going on around the ward, watching patients and staff. One day I heard familiar, loud, high-pitched sounds and looked in the direction they were coming from. I saw a patient, an old man, small in stature. He was unkempt, had a scraggly beard, and fit the stereotypical picture of 'crazy.' The patient was making hand gestures and arm motions while holding a coffee mug, trying to communicate with the ward orderly. The orderly was becoming all the more frustrated with him.

As I watched the interaction, it was obvious to me that the old man was using sign language. He was deaf! He was trying to communicate with the orderly, using his coffee mug asking where to get soap so he could shave. I walked over to the two of them and began signing to the old man. He shrieked with glee and began furiously signing, trying to tell me about wanting to shave, and desperately telling me his story of how he came to be on the ward.

After talking with him, I calmed him down and reassured him I was going to investigate the matter. I read his medical record and immediately realized what was happening. The old man was homeless. He was found on the streets by the police and when they could not communicate with him, they got frustrated. He got scared.

Not all deaf people are mute, they can make sounds but their sounds are odd, if not bizarre, because they have never heard the human voice. The deaf do not know how to gauge their voice, their pitch, or tone. However, they do see the reactions of hearing people in response to their voice; so they remain mute most of the time. However, when they become excited they make noises, and those unfamiliar with them might say they do sound like 'crazy people.'

When the police approached the man, he could not communicate. The cops thought his behavior odd and they took him into custody. When they grabbed him, he became all the more excited and afraid. He began making those bizarre noises louder and louder. The police took the old man to the emergency holding area at the local jail, where he was held overnight. He stood before a judge the next morning.

Due to the old man's inability to communicate, added to the police report, as well as his physical appearance in court, the judge ordered the old man probated. This meant that the man was being placed in the psychiatric hospital for a 90-day evaluation to determine his mental capacity and whether he is a hazard to self or society. The man was locked up in a mental hospital because he was deaf!

I brought the situation to the attention of my instructor. She explained it to the supervisor who mentioned it to the physician. We also discovered the patient's laboratory work had been overlooked. He had diabetes and heart failure. I was instrumental in the man being transferred from a locked mental ward to a nursing home. I often encounter opportunities when my knowledge of sign language and my compassion makes life better for another person.

CHAPTER 63

LOOKING FOR STEPHEN

BY LOIS FINELLI

Who is Stephen?

What makes a person, anyway? Physiology, genes, environment? Or the sum of experience, our history? What happens if we lose ourselves? If we are struck by illness, and can't remember things from our past? What happens if a whole part of ourselves, twenty years of our lifetime, is gone. Are we lost, like a ship without a captain? Once adrift, can the ship still make the same voyage? Or, do we remake ourselves? Are we the same person?

So, who is Stephen?

Stephen says he is from New York, but no one is sure. He could be. That accent—maybe New York, maybe New England, or New Jersey. It's still a mystery.

You see, Stephen never really existed. Not according to Social Security, not according to the FBI, not according to anyone other than Stephen himself. And to us, the County Department of Mental Health, the providers of care.

Of course, he exists. He is living and breathing before us.

Stephen has furnished names, dates, and places. But we have no luck. We cannot find anyone that can tell us more about him. We can find no family, no friends. Just a little information from his chart, just a short year or two ago when he became a Ward of the State, a patient in the mental health system.

So, who was Stephen?

A child raised by nuns, shunned by his parents? A disciple of The Home of Little Wanderers? That's who he says he was.

Stephen says now that he is twenty-four years old and that he was born in 1977. But that doesn't even add up right. Besides, Stephen looks at least sixty.

And he remembers old westerns and old horror films. He can name the actors. (The original Dracula, Bela Lugosi, is his favorite.) We have all accepted that Stephen's birthday is in August, but we can't agree on a year.

His chart gives the diagnosis of Schizophrenia. But Stephen doesn't quite fit that diagnosis. Stephen is different. His uniqueness has fostered the respect of puzzled physicians. Is it schizophrenia? For reimbursement purposes and for Stephen's benefits, having a diagnosis makes life easier for everyone. So be it. But his symptoms and his actions cause uncertainty.

Off medication, Stephen had been known to assume dramatic and some-times macabre poses on the psychiatric ward, or on facility lawns. Once, he was loud and belligerent, gesturing and conversing as if he were the leader of a motorcycle gang. He also became paranoid and suspicious. On medication, though, Stephen is decidedly subdued. But he can still be surreptitious—an escape artist of sorts.

You have to watch Stephen, or he may wander off. Once out of the mental institution, his tenure at other group homes was consistently brief. He didn't want to stay and he couldn't stay. Stephen had places to go. He'd walk out quickly and fervently, with a firm destination in mind.

Stephen had a bad case of wanderlust. Milwaukee, New Brunswick, Hal-loween-town—these are places that Stephen still talks about going, but not as often as before. You see, Stephen is beginning to settle, now that he has lived in our group home. This home is intensive. Lots of staff are available to cater to his individual needs. His need for adventure, his inclination for dressing up and posing are honored. His need for romance is acknowledged. Perhaps the wanderlust is fading away. Maybe he's begun to find what he's been looking for.

Stephen, a budding actor, has played the king in *Sleeping Beauty*. Actually, he did more than play. Stephen metamorphosed into the king. Stephen recited and practiced his lines from *Sleeping Beauty* long after the last curtain call.

Initially, it was difficult for Stephen to put aside his life as king to become the emperor. But he has done just that, with the opportunity to take part in another play, *The Emperor's New Clothes*. He has even grown a beard for the part.

Stephen goes to the ranch once a week. At first, to earn his riding lesson, he cleaned out horse stalls. But, Social Security finally agreed to recognize Stephen as a person deserving of benefits, even without a firm identity. So now, Stephen pays for his weekly riding lesson. His face, usually expression-less, and his voice, usually monotone, convey excitement when he discusses the horses. He lights up. "I sure love those horses!" he once exclaimed, as he talked about his day at the ranch.

So, who is Stephen now?

Stephen's memory is impaired, time has been lost, but nonetheless, small drips and dribbles occur. Some of the past leaks out. Stephen can't help but be reminded of things he has experienced.

Stephen remembers that he slept in train stations and wood sheds. When homeless, he recalls, someone hit him in the mouth and knocked out his teeth. Stephen remembers the name of a devoted nun who took him under her wing during his childhood.

Some things, it is certain, Stephen has never forgotten. Clearly, he is a lover of classical music. Schubert and Mozart are favorites. He identifies the poster of Michelangelo's *The Creation*, over his bed, without hesitation.

Stephen says that he wants a little white mouse to take care of. I wonder about this and recall a conversation I had with him about a grand coach with horses. Could Stephen be thinking about Cinderella's coach, transformed magically from a pumpkin? It was driven by white mice who turned into white horses. Or is this notion my own, evoked by sympathy for Stephen, and spurred on by my appreciation for romance and mystery?

What distinguishes reality from fantasy, or fantasy from imagination? How do we recreate ourselves if we can't remember who we once were?

So, who is Stephen?

Once, he was homeless. Now, he is the emperor, the king, a devoted Catholic, a lover of animals, large and small, and of music, romance, and adventure. Is Stephen a believer in fantasy? Or is he only searching, hopeful that he will meet someone or something familiar?

We know that Stephen is evolving, and that he is gaining strength. You could say that he is reboarding his ship. Twenty-four years are behind him. The course may be uncertain, but the sails are full.

CHAPTER 64

THE CHRISTMAS TREE LADY

BY MARILYN FLETCHER

It was one of those incidents that make you take another look at your life and your world. I picked up the telephone one spring morning in our busy emergency department and heard a young female voice ask, "What should I do with my Christmas trees?"

"I beg your pardon?" was my first response. It had been months since Christmas!

"I have two Christmas trees upstairs and I don't know what to do with them."

Thinking fire hazard, I told her to set them outside on the curb and the town would pick them up. She thanked me and hung up. Half an hour later we received a call from the local police. They were bringing in a young woman who had placed her two toddlers out on the curbside. She said that that's what the hospital told her to do.

When she arrived, the young woman, in her late teens, was obviously confused. Her speech was a constant flow of unrelated ideas. In the middle of her monologue, however, she stopped, looked at me and asked, "Aren't you Jill's mother?"

I answered, "yes." She said that she and Jill went to school together. But before I could pursue that path, she returned to her confused state. Her husband was located at his work and was astounded to see her condition. She had been fine when he left that morning.

She admitted to no medical problems. After a brief physical exam by the doctor, the psychiatric team was called in for an evaluation. The young woman was sent to a psychiatric facility for further care. The children were taken home by their father.

For me, it normally would have ended there, with just the memory of her one lucid moment when she asked about my daughter. But one afternoon, two weeks later, my 15-year-old daughter came home from next door and asked if she could walk to the store to get a pack of cigarettes for the girl who was staying with our neighbors. She explained that the girl had just been released from the hospital and her husband wouldn't let her come home. She ended up next door because she worked with Mrs. Ross, our next-door neighbor, at the nursing home. I looked over to see my 'Christmas Tree Lady' sitting on the porch steps. Startled, I waved at the young woman and said to my daughter, "Sure, go ahead."

A week later, the young woman was gone. I asked my daughter if she had returned home. The answer is frozen in my memory. "Mrs. Ross took her to the doctor's because she was bleeding a lot. She has cancer in her uterus and they say it spread to her brain."

A month later, her obituary was in the paper. The 'what ifs' and 'should haves' have haunted me ever since. It's a story I repeat every time I see someone about to fall through the cracks.

CHAPTER 65

JUST ANOTHER DAY IN THE EMERGENCY ROOM

BY DENISE CASAUBON

It was just another day in the emergency department of a level one trauma center. A Tuesday night filled with car accidents, gun shot wounds, abdominal pain, fevers, and lacerations. It was now early in the morning and the activity was starting to die down.

Another nurse and I were discussing what still needed to be done for the patients that remained in our area: urine collection, a scan of the abdomen, administration of pain medication. We were suddenly interrupted by the charge nurse. We were getting a 21-year-old male complaining of "rat poop" that he couldn't wash off of his body. We looked at each other and simultaneously said, "Room 8." You see, Room 8 is reserved for the patients with psychiatric issues.

The paramedics dutifully brought the patient to us. We didn't know much about him. We were given his name, age, and a brief history of the events that led to his arrival in the emergency department. He was seeing rats and they were pooping on him. His parents had called to have him taken to the hospital because the young man had taken at least ten showers at home.

Before I entered the room, I stopped and said a silent prayer. "Please Lord, give me wisdom and give me strength. Do not let any harm come to either one of us." Before me was a naked young man whose eyes darted to all corners of the room. His head jerked quickly, then he ducked. I could feel my eyebrows wrinkle up. This guy had some very bad drugs on board. Softly, I called his name and asked him to look at me. When I had his attention, I asked him what was wrong. He replied, "All the rats are pooping on me. Can I please take a shower?"

"No, no shower," I said. I obtained what history I could. The patient admitted to smoking marijuana. I went to talk to the resident caring for this patient. Security was called to sit with him in case the patient wanted to harm himself or others.

When I returned to the room moments later, the patient announced he had to go to the bathroom. Excellent! I needed to get a urine sample to send for a drug screen. I got a gown on him and we walked past three other patients' beds on the way to the bathroom. Even though I assured him there were no rats in the hospital, we were dodging those darn rats the entire way to the bathroom.

Within two seconds, I realized my mistake. I had taken him to use the only bathroom with a shower. He was undressed and had the water on before I could close the bathroom door. He was spraying the water so much that my feet got wet. I sternly told him to finish washing and get out of the shower. I yelled for security to bring me towels and a new gown. Needless to say, I did not obtain any urine. We marched back to his room together in silence.

Apparently, the security guard fell for the same story, because less than ten minutes later, I was getting my second shower of the morning. This time, though, the patient was bobbing and ducking like the rats were jumping off the walls at him. I was afraid he was going to fall in the wet shower and hurt himself. I remained calm. I offered reassurance. I allowed him one minute to shower. Then I made him get out and dry off. Again, we trudged back to his room past the other three patients.

Finally an order came for sedative medications. They were greatly needed. The only challenge would be administering two intermuscular injections to this patient. Myself and another RN went into the room. The rats were apparently also on the floor, so the patient decided to jump up on the gurney. And he would not stand still. I am sure to anyone unaware of the situation, I am the one that sounded psychotic: "Dude, sit down. Let me have your butt, I have to give you a shot. There are no rats in the room. Please sit down."

We were not getting anywhere. Then I had a thought. If he allowed us to give the medication, I would allow him to take one more shower. Yes, I promised. Thankfully, he got into a kneeling position on the gurney. On the count of three the shots were over. On four, we were off to the shower, again. This time, I went willingly. After a short shower and the most vigorous towel drying I have ever seen someone give themselves, we were back to his room. Warm blankets and a pillow were offered. The lights were turned out. The security officer was in his place. Within minutes, the patient was asleep.

He may not remember that morning. In a way I hope that he doesn't. I could see how tortured he was by looking into his eyes. But part of me prays that he does remember, so that he will never use drugs again. Next time, the angels may not be watching over him.

CHAPTER 66

NEW MOM

BY AQUILLA T. MILLER AND DEBBIE DULANEY

I once read that nurses are God's special helpers, and as far as I am concerned, this is true. We are telling our story of how Debby, my nurse, and I, a pregnant, first-time mom-to-be met and the magic that followed. Once the clinic confirmed that I was indeed 12 weeks pregnant, I was referred to a program for first-time mothers. After filling out a lot of paperwork, I was admitted to the program. The program lasted two years and a nurse would visit you in your home to teach about the different stages of pregnancy and child development.

This is when Debby entered my life. She came to visit and would bring worksheets, books, and videos to increase my knowledge about pregnancy. She was extremely patient and a good listener. I did my best to use the information Debby gave me. She made a huge impact on my expectations about childbirth, decreasing the horror stories I had heard from other women.

I was fortunate to have no complications during my pregnancy. Indeed, I had only two episodes of morning sickness. My husband had more morning sickness than me. We ate a lot of Saltines. Debby also had worksheets and questionnaires for him. As he worked with these, he became more involved in becoming a father. Working with Debby helped both of us realize what we had to contribute to our growing family.

I couldn't get over how comfortable I was with Debby and we became real friends. I was familiar with many of the things the baby would need and so I learned quickly. I enjoyed Debby's easy style and her willingness to answer my questions. I felt God had sent me an angel. As I got closer to delivery, I saw Debby a bit less, as I needed time to get myself and the house prepared.

Early in my pregnancy, the due date was uncertain. Once I met my doctor, however, he told me the date would be February 24, 2001. He was right. On that day, I gave birth to a seven pound, seven ounce boy.

Then I got to show off what I had learned from Debby. I am sure the delivery room staff would not have told me my baby's Apgar score, if I hadn't asked. The staff wanted to know where I learned about an Apgar score. My answer, of course, was my wonderful nurse. The staff was very impressed!

After returning home with our son Jairus, I couldn't wait for Debby to see him. She was so good with Jairus. I was amazed to learn that Debby was not a mother herself. She was such a passionate caregiver for babies. She taught me about how babies grow and what to expect in general terms. Babies are so different that you can't expect them to grow "by the book." Jairus was very unpredictable and it took me some time to accept that he was OK, just growing according to his own timetable. Debby taught me to celebrate progress and not to get upset when Jairus did not do what I expected.

I was sad when Jairus turned two. I thought I might lose touch with Debby. The program ended, but not my relationship with Debby. She continued to be my friend and to be there for us. I am amazed at how she goes into stranger's homes, some of which are not clean and neat, and brings order and knowledge. When I questioned Debby about the safety of going into a stranger's home, she assured me no one has ever been disrespectful or negative. It just takes time to know people. I was always taught to count your blessings no matter what the circumstances. I always count Debby twice! Angels do come around.

CHAPTER 67

INTENSIVE CARING

BY TERESA JULICH

Lois, a 70-year-old woman, was brought to the medical ICU where I was a nurse, with multiple abscesses on her spine and around her lungs which were causing severe infection throughout her entire body. As the days passed Lois's chances of survival looked more and more bleak. Lois was only minimally responsive and she needed a ventilator to breathe for her. Therefore, she was unable to make her own decisions about the healthcare that she received. She had no living will, so we carried on as a healthcare team to provide her the best care possible until her family could be reached to make decisions for her.

Lois's eldest daughter, Darlene, was called and made aware of the situation early on, but she lived many hours away. She arranged to be at her mother's side as quickly as she could. She would ultimately be responsible for her mother's care and she would be the decision-maker—a task she was very uneasy about taking on.

Darlene remained at her mother's side 24 hours a day praying and talking, hoping for the best. Week after week went by and Lois showed little signs of improvement. The infection inside her body was slowly killing her. Darlene was not doing well. She was not eating or sleeping because she was constantly worrying about her mother. In her mind, she should not be the one who decided to let her mother live or die. If only the responsibility didn't rest of her shoulders, it would have been much easier for her to deal with. Day after day, she fought an internal battle within herself. She didn't want her mother to suffer, but she didn't want to be the one who gave up hope either.

One evening while caring for Lois, I heard Darlene crying in the corner of her mother's room. I waited a few minutes to let Darlene grieve and then I entered the room to attempt to comfort her. I sat down next to her in silence, putting my hand on her shoulder. After a few quiet moments, Darlene looked at me and said, "Is your mom still living?" I hesitated a minute wondering where this question was leading. I remembered that I was taught in nursing school to never discuss your own problems with the patients or their families. Use therapeutic communication, the professors used to say.

"No," I finally answered with tears in my eyes. "She was killed when I was 18 years old." Darlene's eyes got big as she looked up at me. She had a look of relief on her face. Finally there was someone who might understand what she was dealing with. We continued talking. I told her about how tough it is to lose a mother or someone you love but also how it has changed my life in a positive way. I shared stories of my mother with her and we even laughed together. After about 15 minutes of sharing memories there was silence again. Darlene grabbed my hand and gave it a tight squeeze. She looked at me and said, "Thank you." We hugged and I began to walk out of the room. As I was about to leave, she said, "I think I'm finally ready." Darlene was ready to let her mother rest and be at peace.

Early the next morning with Darlene at her side, Lois passed away peacefully and without pain. Darlene was overwhelmed by sadness but felt at peace with the decision she was making for her mother and the rest of the family. As nurses, we get so busy sometimes that we forget to just sit and talk to patients and their families. Darlene just needed some support and someone to listen to her thoughts in order to make the best decision for her mother. Many times it takes days or hours to make tough decisions like these but sometimes it only takes a moment of sharing.

Chapter 68

Bernard

By Teresa Lynn Greeson

The night shift began as all the rest. A hurried report given by the day nurse who was eager to get home after a long 12-hour shift in the emergency department. "The patient in Bed 3 is a 92-year-old man who came in for right lower quadrant pain while having a bowel movement. He has a history of an abdominal aortic aneurysm with repair. He's in CT-scan now, and Dr. Zinn is with him." The red flag automatically went up; this is serious.

When Bernard came back from the scan, we knew the news was bad. Dr. Z immediately ordered a consult with the vascular surgeon on call. We overheard the conversation. The aneurysm had ruptured.

The surgeon arrived, reviewed the films and radiologist's report. He then asked me to join him when he spoke to the patient and his family. "Mr. Simons, your aneurysm has ruptured again. You are bleeding into your abdominal cavity, and there's nothing we can do. I can't operate. You are going to die from this. All we can do is make you comfortable." He said the words so matter-of-factly, as if he were giving him a stock market report. "I'm sorry. There's nothing we can do." The doctor left the room, leaving us all in a stunned silence.

Bernard's daughter was called in New York. We put a telephone in his room so that he could talk to her. "Peg—it's bad. We have to say goodbye. I love you. I have to tell you goodbye." I have never heard such heartbreaking words. As my eyes filled with tears, I left the room to cry, thinking of my own parents, and thanking God that they were still here with me.

As the hours passed, Bernard became restless. The blood pooling in his abdomen pressed on his diaphragm, making it harder to breathe. We hung a morphine drip; it helped, Bernard said. I sat alone at his bedside for an hour, wiping the sweat off his face, giving him sips of water, and lubricating his lips. "Are you comfortable?" I asked. "Oh, I make a living," he jokingly replied. In his dying hours, Bernard still managed a smile, and told me "you're a swell bunch."

His girlfriend entered the room, her eyes red and swollen from crying. As she kissed his forehead, he repeated the same gut-wrenching words. "We have to say goodbye." I left them alone to share their last moments together, and to hide in the break room to cry. I collected myself and went back to Bernard offering a cool rag for his forehead, another sip of water. "Are you comfortable?" "I make a living." His sister came in, and again, he said those words. "We have to say goodbye."

His girlfriend went home, kissing him goodbye and saying, "I love you. You are my Prince Charming." So began my night-long vigil—wiping his brow, moistening his lips, increasing the morphine when Bernard became restless and uncomfortable. His sister stayed all night, sitting, watching, and waiting for the end to come. At 7:20 AM, I gave report to the day nurse, amazed that he had survived the night. I went back to Bernard's room to tell his sister goodbye. She thanked me over and over for all that I had done for her, and for her brother. Bernard was now comatose, heavily medicated with morphine, and breathing the slow, deep gasps that I've come to recognize as those of the dying. As Bernard's sister talked, I watched his heart rate drop from 72 to 59. Then 40s, then 30s. Then 18. I interrupted her. "It's time. You need to tell him goodbye, and let him know it's okay to go." She looked at me, eyes wide with the shock of knowing that Bernard was, at that very moment, dying. "I can't say goodbye. Is it really time?"

"Yes. You have to say goodbye now. He needs to know that it's okay to go."

She kissed his forehead and cheek, whispering in his ear that it was okay to go, and how much she loved him. She kissed his face as I watched his heart rate continue to slow... 18... 10... 6... 0. He was gone.

A rare opportunity was given to me this night. As an RN of only two months, I was still working with my preceptor. Because of her, I was able to stay with Bernard all night, while she took care of our other patients. I was able to sit with him, wiping the sweat from his face, holding his hand, and helping him leave this life for what lies beyond.

The 12 and one-half hours that I spent with Bernard and his family broke my heart. Hearing him say goodbye to his daughter, sister, and girlfriend was the saddest thing I've ever experienced in all my years of working in the medical field. But I also know how fortunate I was; fortunate to have met Bernard and to have made his last hours peaceful, painless, and comfortable.

On this night, the most special night of my career, I helped Bernard die.

Chapter 69

The Essence of Nursing

By Marge McDowell
and
J.M. Pantatello

John was one of those people whose spirit shone through his eyes. You could always tell what John was really feeling by just looking at his blue eyes.

John was a retired high school principal who had been in a car accident and suffered a hip injury as well as internal bleeding. The hip repair had to wait while the internal bleeding was repaired. As a result, the physician worried about the hip becoming necrotic which would not allow John to bear any weight. John was recovering from his injuries, but was having a very difficult time being weaned from the ventilator. He'd had polio when he was younger and the physicians suspected post-polio weakness of the muscles of respiration. Weaning and walking were a real trial for John. When he got up with the walker, he had to deal with shortness of breath, fear, and our constant reminders not to put any weight on his right leg. I've never seen anyone work so hard on his rehabilitation. He tried so hard to do everything right, and would become easily discouraged with himself.

One day we were helping John walk to the door of his room. The stress of the activity, together with the tube feedings he was receiving, combined to cause plops of diarrhea stool to fall out onto the floor. I quickly wiped it up, hoping John hadn't noticed. No chance. We continued the walk. When John finally got back to bed, he looked at me with those blue eyes and then covered his face with his hands in a gesture of total shame.

John was a sensitive man, and I had the strong feeling that this was an important interaction between us. It seemed as if his spirit desperately needed the right words to keep him from giving up. How could I give him what he needed without sounding superficial or phony? I knew that those eyes would catch on in a minute if I didn't mean what I was saying. I took a deep breath and thought about what I would need to hear if I was the one in the bed. It seemed right to explain to him that we all knew him as a person of incredible strength and dignity, and that our knowledge of him as a person came from working with him day by day and seeing his determination and struggle. I told him that what had just happened was a physical thing that had nothing to do with him as a person. I explained that he did not need to be ashamed of something that meant nothing to us. These words seemed to hang in mid air for a minute as he searched my eyes. Then he relaxed ever so slightly and mouthed, "Thank you."

There are so many occasions like this that may seem insignificant at first. When we take the time to be where the patient is and reach inside ourselves to give what is needed, we just might make the difference between fighting on and giving up. It takes effort to be where the patient is, to be able to read their eyes, but it's part of the essence of nursing.

Chapter 70

Special Person

By Patricia A. Layton

In September 1991 my daughter was in a terrible car accident. She was two years old. She was strapped in her car seat in the middle of the back seat. I was at work that day. A co-worker told me that my daughter was in an accident and drove me to the hospital. As we passed the car on the way to the emergency room, I couldn't believe that anyone could have survived the accident. The car was totaled. I knew where my daughter's car seat was sitting and that part of the car was all caved in.

I arrived at the hospital to find my daughter laughing in a nurse's arms. She was bleeding from her head and had a broken leg. The nurse put her in a whirlpool bath to get the blood and glass off of her. She said, "I went for a swim, Mommy." As I waited for the doctor to stitch her head and set her leg, I would check on my husband who was in the next room, also with head injuries.

I remember a male nurse who held my daughter and made her laugh, while I ran back and forth from room to room. He cared about me and he cared about my family. I decided that day, that I would become a nurse, too. I just couldn't forget the nurse who cared so much.

Today, I am a Registered Nurse in an emergency department. When things get hectic, I think of the male nurse who made such a difference in my life. I just wish I had the chance to let him know what he meant to me and my family. My whole world changed that day. Thank you to the nurse who cared so much.

CHAPTER 71

PURDY DARN GOOD PUBLIC HEALTH NURSE

BY KATE BRACY KALB

It would be easy to write off Lydia Morgan. At age 28 she has been pregnant six times. During each pregnancy she used some combination of alcohol, crack cocaine, and heroine. She has five living children, none of whom are allowed to live with her.

Enter Diana, public health nurse with Moms Plus, a program that works with substance abusing pregnant women. Diana met Lydia during her second trimester at an inpatient treatment center in Seattle. "I've been very impressed with Lydia because it is so clear how much she wants this baby, and how much she *doesn't* want history to repeat itself," Diana tells me as we drive into a residential area. I am working on an article for our health department newsletter, so Diana is taking me as a "ride along."

"She is trying to get her baby back home, and is living in 'transitional housing' until she and Bill can find a more stable place." Diana speaks of Lydia with great fondness, describing her as "talkative and honest, warm and lively." She tells me I will find Lydia charming. I cast her a dubious glance, thinking about the woman's history. She throws me a 'you'll see' smile and points to a piece of paper in the back seat, which I pick up. In careful calligraphy it says, "Purdy Darn Good Public Health Nurse Award. Thanx!" She explains that Lydia's partner, Bill, made it for her. She tells me Bill has been a constant support for Lydia, and she has enjoyed watching them develop as a couple. She plans to frame the calligraphy for her office.

We pull up in front of a rundown house, with a dry patch of weeds serving as a front yard. As we go down the side path to the back door, Diana knocks on a basement window, and says, "That's her cue that I'm here." We are greeted from the tiny back porch by an exuberant Lydia. She is small, red-headed, and obviously delighted to see Diana. "Guess what? Guess what?" she hugs Diana, and briefly shakes my hand. "Bill is working full time!"

"That's wonderful!" Diana replies, as we are led past closed doors to a small living room–bed room combination, with a double bed, a large maple console television, a coffee table, and two chairs. The carpet is worn, but clean. In an alcove, an empty white crib is visible, with several plastic bags of baby things under it. Lydia motions for us to take the chairs, and offers us a cup of coffee.

Lydia knows why I'm here and is happy to talk to me about herself and the Moms Plus program. For the next hour she sits on the floor across from me, and we chat about who she is, how she got here, and where she is going. It is not an easy tale.

"Being clean and sober now, I really regret using drugs in my pregnancies," she says. "I'm losing out on five children's lives today. They don't even want to write me." She pauses briefly, tears welling, then continues, "I caused them pain. I caused them hurt. They have not had a mother for years."

She goes on to describe many attempts at treatment, including two unsuccessful attempts during this last pregnancy. Finally, she says, she managed to complete three consecutive 26-day inpatient treatment sessions by finishing one, and then checking herself back in the next day, saying "I'm getting the urge to use." This was the only way she could maintain sobriety through the end of her pregnancy.

"I know it doesn't look good on paper, checking back in like that, but I never relapsed." She says it proudly. She has been clean for six months.

I ask her to tell me about her children. She responds rapidly, "Natalie, Elise, Abbey. One's in Montana, one is in Idaho, one's in Oregon — adopted. Esteban was up for adoption too, he's gone. With Jasmine I had a miscarriage. Amanda is the one in Idaho. I got an open adoption with her. And now Angelica. Angelica Hope Lydia Morgan Garcia."

I try to absorb the sheer multitude of this response. I ask what is different about this most recent baby. She brightens.

"This baby changed my life. I have her and a man I'd die for. Those two, that's my sobriety right there." She pauses to consider, "I think Child Protection Services (CPS) wants her, but with God as my witness, I will not let them get her. I want one of my kids with me. I didn't name my baby 'Hope' for nothing! There's a reason that little girl is here right now."

I ask both of them about what have been the hardest moments. Diana answers first, "It was really hard when CPS came to the hospital. It was the same worker who took her last baby."

Lydia interrupts, "Five hours after I gave birth, CPS came and snagged her. That was wrong because I did everything I could to maintain my sobriety. I still am doing everything I can. You give birth to a healthy baby, a clean baby and, pow, they come and take her. How am I going to show you guys that I can be a mother to this baby if you don't let me bring her home?"

She continues, very animated now, "I don't care if you sit across from my house for a year! Let me have a chance with my baby."

Though intense, she speaks with confidence. Her words sound positive, and not angry as much as enthusiastic. She hands me a picture of a gorgeous red-faced newborn with dark tousled hair. Somehow I find myself believing her.

Diana adds, "She was really devastated because she'd been clean, and the baby was clean, so she thought it would be different from last time." Lydia listens quietly as Diana describes working with her. "I think Lydia really responds well to emotional support. She needs people around who see her best side, and when you do that, she rallies." Lydia is smiling, nodding as she listens.

I ask Lydia what it's been like for her to have Moms Plus involved in her life. "Well, I never had no one with me in my other pregnancies. I've got quite a bit of support with this one. And the Moms Plus workers are confidential. I don't have much trust in people, but I trust Diana one hundred percent. I can talk to her anytime about my serious situations, good or bad. It makes me feel relief."

In the course of the interview, I watch Diana work. When Lydia hesitates, she smiles encouragement. At one point we are interrupted by a call from Lydia's sister in St. Paul. She is flying in tomorrow with her daughter. "Oh yes, do come!" Lydia says excitedly. I look around the tiny room wondering where two extra people could possibly stay. Diana helps her think through getting to the airport on the bus, and suggests arranging for her sister to join her when she visits the baby. Later, when Lydia is talking about not having any teeth (something that never bothered her when she was using drugs) Diana suggests a goal of getting an appointment at the university dental clinic for dentures. Lydia smiles at me, saying, "See! That's what Moms Plus is all about. They help you with everything!"

I ask what the plan is now for Lydia. Together Lydia and Diana go over the list. First there will be neuro-psychological testing next month. Then Lydia will have to get into a treatment program, start mental health counseling, and find parenting classes. She and Bill must have drug-free urine tests throughout the evaluation period and beyond. Both women speak comfortably, as though success is not only possible but probable. They discuss places for treatment. I see the hope in Lydia's face and hear it in her tone. Diana's cheerful, soothing voice reassures her as they talk. They could be friends going over plans for a first dinner party. I realize that Diana was right. I *am* charmed. I want this to work

Later, I ask Diana what it's like to work with people like Lydia, and why would she choose this particular career. She responds without hesitation, "To me it feels like a miracle. I have so much faith in the power of recovery. It's a privilege and honor to be a part of that with a patient. It's like watching them move from a darkened corridor onto a path of light. You watch them leave behind the pain and addiction and abuse."

She talks about the admission process, "The initial intake is more than an intake, it is an opportunity. It is very powerful hearing a client's stories. People break down and cry and talk about when they were using. It's a poignant time. It bonds you. And from there you can put together a powerful package of services to support them."

"Look at Lydia," she continues, "I've seen her tenderly try to pick herself up. It's lovely, and clumsy. It may only happen two or three times a year that someone does this well, out of maybe 50 clients. But it's so powerful when it does happen. You just know that you have to give everyone a chance."

"I mean, think about it. How do you figure out what to do with your life when you've been so lost for so long? It's an honor to watch them be people they have never been before, to be one of their helping hands. It's a spiritual thing, really."

It *is* a spiritual thing. I heard it in her calm voice as she reminded Lydia that baby Hope would remember her touch, even if she could only visit three days a week. I watched it in her accepting gaze and the warm looks that passed between them, and noted it in the optimistic way she described Lydia's chances of being a good mom. I felt it as the room came alive with Lydia's sad stories and growing hopes.

It is a spiritual thing indeed. And "purdy darn good" public health nursing to boot.

CHAPTER 72

CHANGING MY LIFE'S DIRECTION

BY LENORE B. WEINSTEIN

Never in my wildest dreams did I ever imagine that I would go from being a practicing nurse to working with eyewitnesses of the Holocaust, primarily survivors. Who would have thought that my nursing career track would take such a unique direction? Or that my nursing background would be helpful in preparing me for this meaningful new role and worthwhile endeavor.

As a new graduate nurse, I worked in maternity, labor and delivery, newborn nursery, and newborn intensive care. I then taught community health nursing, supervised nursing students in home health care, and worked with families and older adults. Working with the elderly may have been a contributing factor in my interest and ability to work with Holocaust survivors and other eyewitnesses. Later on, I was involved with school health projects and research in gerontology. So, how did it come about that I am currently working in Holocaust education and with Holocaust eyewitnesses?

Applications and contests in newspapers and magazines—I'm constantly filling out forms. Little did I know that an application that I completed almost ten years ago regarding interest in working with Holocaust eyewitnesses would change my life and impact me in the most far-reaching manner. I was invited to attend an interviewer training seminar where I learned history, research, and interviewer techniques. I watched documentaries, videos, heard lectures and participated in discussions with Holocaust survivors and other eyewitnesses. Upon completing the training seminar, I was certified to interview Holocaust survivors and other eyewitnesses. I then attended a college-accredited interviewer training course that worked with Holocaust documentation and education, and received their certification enabling me to interview and participate in Holocaust education.

There are several aspects to my Holocaust work, but the one closest to my heart and which offers me the greatest challenge and satisfaction is conducting videotaped interviews with Holocaust eyewitnesses, primarily survivors. Hearing the eyewitnesses' testimony is difficult. Even though it happened over 55 years ago, the pain is still fresh. The stories are horrific—one cannot believe the level of man's inhumanity to man.

Over the past ten years, I have interviewed, or rather, heard testimony from, almost 250 Holocaust survivors, liberators, refugees, saviors, and rescuers. I have heard about people's lives before, during, and since World War II and the Holocaust. People I have interviewed have suffered involuntary relocation, deportations, been in ghettoes, hid in underground places as well as under assumed names and identities with false papers, fought as partisans, were part of other resistance groups, experienced miraculous escapes, were prisoners in labor, concentration, and death camps, survived Death Marches and endured extreme tortures. Most survivors lost part, or all of their families.

I have heard young American soldiers who entered concentration camps and liberated the prisoners without knowing what they would find, describe their trauma. I have listened to brave individuals who risked their and their family members' lives to save others insist that they were not heroes; that it was the 'right thing to do' and they 'only did what needed to be done'. Sometimes it feels as if my heart stops when I hear their stories. I hear accounts of survival, bravery, courage, and the resilience of the human spirit.

The eyewitnesses talk, and I listen while the interview is videotaped, recording historic events and creating a historical document. The work is heartbreaking and challenging. My life has been touched in ways that I couldn't ever imagine. Nothing I have ever done before is comparable. The stories and testimonials that I have listened to are incredible. The interview allows the survivor to give their testimony, providing their history, use elements of storytelling, reminiscence, and the life-review process which provide therapeutic benefits to the teller. Many of my interviewees have told me that they have never talked about this before, especially to their children. But when they are finished, I often hear them say that they are glad that they told their story—so that their children will know, their grandchildren will know, and the world will know.

What an indescribable feeling it is to be part of this, helping them leave a legacy for future generations! This work involves trust, emotions, and the baring of one's soul. A special, often lasting, bond is formed. I have kept in touch over the years with many of the people I have interviewed, through holiday cards, telephone calls, through good and, unfortunately, bad news. I often see many of them at memorial services, programs, and lectures that I attend.

Another aspect of my work is education. I am involved with middle, high school, and university students in full-day, anti-prejudice programs, working with survivors to teach the students about the Holocaust. We also discuss the dangers of hatred and intolerance, and expand their knowledge and understanding of the past. The students describe this "Student Awareness Day" as an experience they will remember for the rest of their lives. The Holocaust survivors frequently describe their satisfaction in sharing their stories with the next generation.

The state of Florida, among other states, has mandated teaching of the Holocaust in secondary school and so I work with the annual Teacher Training Institute and other programs for educators that provide teacher training for this objective. I also help train and evaluate potential interviewers who are seeking certification.

My nurse's training, with the caring and sensitivity that we, as nurses, extend to our patients, has given me a basis to work with Holocaust eyewitnesses. It is no wonder that so many interviewers, and Holocaust educators are nurses and that nurses particularly are successful interviewers of Holocaust survivors.

It has been a privilege and an honor to be the recipient of eyewitness accounts of the Holocaust and to be part of preserving this history for future generations.

Yes, indeed, nurses are everywhere—including in the unique role of Holocaust education and interviewing eyewitnesses to the Holocaust.

CHAPTER 73

LOW'S LEGACY

BY LORRAINE STEEFEL, AS TOLD BY EMMANUEL FALLAH

Emmanuel Fallah had an unlikely education. It wasn't in the formal classrooms of a university, although he was an International Relations student at the University of Monrovia, Liberia. His classroom was the bush country of a land at war. It was 1996 during the climax of the then seven-year-old civil war that first sent his native land into chaos. There were no pens or paper. He was on the road, traversing his country on foot, fleeing Monrovia, Liberia's capital, for his life.

When the American embassy wouldn't accept him and his friend Oliver, Emmanuel chose the alternative, to walk the opened corridor, some 300 miles south toward the Ivory Coast border. Late in the evening some two days later, they were lost, searching for villagers who might know the way toward the next town, when they came across three women. "Don't kill us," they begged. "We're just like you," Emmanuel and Oliver told them. "We're trying to make our way to the border."

"We're following this woman who knows the way. Join us," one of the women said. So a friendship of convenience that developed into a family was born—three women, two men, later joined by a few others. They were a tightly knit group who didn't dare divulge their last names or occupations. These were suspicious times. Last names revealed your tribe, where you came from. Occupations revealed whether or not you worked for the government. Either could cause you to be killed should this information fall into rebel hands.

Lowella, affectionately called Low, was the leader of the group. Emmanuel was soon to discover much about this tall, lighter-complexioned, 40-year old woman. She was a descendant of Americo-Liberians, freed American slaves who established Liberia in 1820. Low was a nurse, a graduate of Cuttington University's nursing program in Suacocco, a city in central Liberia. Her identification card said that she worked as a nurse administrator at JFK Medical Center, the largest, most sophisticated government-run hospital in the country. To protect herself, Low disguised herself. She kept her long black hair tied up under a short curly haired wig.

For two days, the group foraged for food by day and slept whenever and wherever night caught up with them. Gunfire hedged in on them. It was normal to walk past people dying from starvation or illness in the bush—a wide-eyed child searching for his mother, an old woman breathing her last breath.

"Help me!" came a piercing cry. But the group walked a few feet away, until Low heard a woman scream. "Nurse, doctor. Somebody, is there a nurse that can help me? My water broke." Low hesitated. "Come on, Low, we have to go on," the group warned. Let's find out what's happening there," Low said.

Hidden in the bush, lying next to the dead body of her six-year old son, a young mother was about to give birth. "We have to help her," Low said. "She might be a rebel or someone wanted by the rebels," the group responded. "Time is of the essence to escape. We can't do anything for her anyway."

"I'm a nurse," Low said. She took off her wig and said, "I can no longer keep up my disguise. If the rebels kill me, whatever happens, happens. We have to help this woman."

Low began giving orders. "Open this can with your penknife," she told Emmanuel. "Empty the fruit and fetch water in the can from the stream. Start a fire and boil the water. Dip your penknife into the boiled water and bring it to me."

Emmanuel watched Low create a make-shift suction device out of a small tube that Low used to carry her keys. He watched Low instruct the mother when to breathe and when to push. He heard the mother's delirious cries to some unseen person. "I agree to die but don't kill my child," she screamed.

Soon the cries of a newborn mingled with the tears and smiles of the new mother. Emmanuel witnessed his first birth and watched as Low cut the umbilical cord with the penknife, suctioned the baby's nose with the hollowed tube, and presented the infant to his mother. "He will be named Courage-Low," said the mother. "Courage because of how he was born and Low after his savior."

Blood began to seep out from the new mother. Low called for the groups' jackets and pressed them against the woman's body to stop the flow. The group tried to convince Low to leave. "She's not going to live. We can't carry her. We can't take care of her or the baby." The decision wasn't theirs to make. A still, lifeless body with unseeing eyes told them to take her child and move on.

Low carried the infant, wondering what to feed it "I have no breast milk. What am I to do?" Emmanuel heard her say. Low cut her fingernails short and pressed down the back of the baby's tongue, carefully feeding it small drops of boiled stream water. The baby survived.

Low had a beaming smile that exposed a wide space between her teeth. When she spoke, she used her hands to emphasize a point. During the next two days, Low smiled and emphasized many points to Emmanuel. "It was the first time I heard the story of nursing; what it is and its ideals," says Emmanuel. "Low spoke to me about Florence Nightingale's vision to help others. She said that nursing is not an extension of a woman's domestic role although most people in Africa think so."

Low told Emmanuel that she could never have left the pregnant woman. "The minute I saw her, my conscience told me that she was my patient," Low said. "I could never have lived with the guilt had I passed her by."

Low wanted to make a mark, to leave a legacy. She believed that nurses can make a difference. She, as a nurse, wanted to run for a seat in the government. This is how she believed she could create change for nursing as a respected career and for her country that was in such dire straits.

"Do you agree with me about how we can make a change in the government?" Low asked Emmanuel. "But you're fighting an uphill battle in Africa where you fear for your life," Emmanuel answered. "But I can make a change as a nurse. Think about it," she said.

After a few minutes, Low asked, "Do you believe that a single person can make a change?" "Most likely," Emmanuel said. "But do you believe me?" she asked.

"Yes," Emmanuel said. "Then say it out loud. Say, I can make a change," Low said.

"I can make a change," Emmanuel said.

Finally the group was nearing a non-government run organization that would receive them as refugees and care for the baby. A rebel checkpoint stood between them and the organization. The men passed through easily but the rebels refused to release two of the women, saying that they were too beautiful to leave. Last was Low carrying the baby. "How is it that you have a baby?" the rebels asked. They interrogated Low until she told them the baby's story and admitted that she was the nurse who delivered him. "Finally, we have a nurse," the rebels said. "You and the baby will go with us to the frontline where you will care for our wounded."

Low pleaded with them to let the baby go. They refused. When one of the female rebels tried to take the infant away from her, she held it tightly and said, "You'll have to kill me first." Emmanuel will never forget Low or the sight of Low being pushed onto the floor of the back of the Toyota pick-up truck. She was crying and waving, holding on to Courage-Low with her life.

By her intervention, Low allowed a refugee mother to see her baby born, saved an infant, led a group to safety, and nurtured a passion for nursing in Emmanuel, now a new graduate nurse, who witnessed her efforts. This is Low's legacy.

CHAPTER 74

THE HEART OF HEALING

BY FRAN NIELSEN

I was trembling and scared as I left the gynecology clinic at the University of Iowa Hospital on July 2, 2002. Only hours before, I felt strong and vigilant about my health and fitness status. My diligence of monthly self breast exams was ongoing. I was there for my yearly checkup—breast and body exams and a pap smear—that all conscientious women schedule, but don't easily anticipate. My gynecologist radiated her usual warmth and compassion, qualities that infused her patients with trust. During a thorough exam she palpated a small lump, the size of a pinhead, at the base of my left breast.

A Registered Nurse for 41 years and having cared for hundreds of breast cancer patients, I knew that a surgical biopsy was the gold standard for a definitive diagnosis. My mammogram and fine needle aspiration specimens proved negative. I had a history of two previous breast biopsies. On both occasions the lumps were benign cysts. On this third experience I was rationally prepared, but still went through the mental process of 'what if.' What if it's positive?

The procedure was done at the surgeon's office and then I returned home to rest and wait. I would receive a call from my doctor in four to five days with the final pathology report. It was a difficult week with preoccupations of malignancy, body alterations, and short life expectancy. To help me focus on positive thoughts I drew strength from God and nature.

July was a beautiful month, bright and sunny, and my fifteen rose bushes were decorated with peach and red flowers against green shiny leaves. It was Friday, the fifth day following my surgical biopsy, and I was getting ready to cut some roses to add color to the dining room table. At 1:00 PM the phone rang and I gently picked the receiver up. I only remember hearing the words "Your biopsy is positive." In that instant, my world fell apart like a 1,000-piece puzzle that I had meticulously put together over a very long time. My masterpiece fell and shattered all over the floor. I didn't know where to start restoring this precious project. I was unable to focus on an approach—by color, by border, by picture—I felt so lost!

I clutched on to my husband to draw strength—my breath, my laughter, my thoughts and dreams for the future all came to a stop. Feeling stunned with a heart filled with pain, Dave and I cried, prayed, and clung to each other not knowing what else to do. We felt helpless.

My surgeon was gentle and kind and gradually gave us all of the information from the pathology report and microscopic analysis. This included tumor size, type, and staging and defined options of treatments. I had to suddenly make decisions from a list of choices I never wanted to make.

I had been a jogger for 32 years, interested in diet and exercise, had assisted physicians, and always was called upon to heal others. Modern medicine allows opportunity to preserve the body and defeat cancer by selecting radiation, chemotherapy, and anti-hormone drugs. Each patient has the right to make his or her choice based on facts, age, physical considerations, function, and what predicted outcome they can best live with. I opted for a bilateral mastectomy, and because of the very small tumor size with no lymph node involvement, I did not require any additional therapies. It was a choice that I could make, with Dave's love and approval, and be okay.

My surgery, post-operative period, and recovery went well. Nursing care was excellent and all hospital staff members were kind, compassionate, and professional. I was surrounded by my family—all of whom have roots in the medical community. My husband directs the physical therapy program at the University of Iowa. Our youngest son and daughter are both physical therapists and our two older sons are medical doctors (a surgeon and an ER/trauma doctor). They all have tender hearts and deep spiritual faith. They filled me with confidence, strength, and support throughout my journey.

I began the healing process and progressively returned to walking three to four miles, jogging, and, with doctor approval, stretching and weight training. My daughter, Kim, designed three creative warm-up and flexibility exercises that I did three times a day. Between her great coaching and my compliance I had a quick and amazing physical recovery. That feeling of regaining control elevated my sense of independence and self-esteem and ignited my passion to return to nursing.

In September, six weeks following my surgery, I returned to 3 West to resume my role of an RN. My first day back went smoothly and staff greeted me warmly. On the second day, things seemed different and difficult when I was assigned three breast cancer patients. I was proficient at teaching them home care of their drainage devices, wound management, and signs and symptoms to report to their physician. On the outside I appeared confident, but on the inside I felt sad and deeply challenged. Emotionally, I felt drained.

I thought that if I was physically strong, in time I would fully heal. After two months I experienced insomnia, but continued to work three to four days per week. With inadequate sleep for my body to recover, I began spiraling downward and had difficulty engaging with others and remembering things. This was a dark time for me. My husband was strong and solid and navigated me to seek medical attention. My internist, a woman of deep compassion, prescribed medication for sleep and depression and referred me to a wonderful psychologist.

This was a new encounter for me and I realized that I had been through a life-altering experience. I would never be the same and it required making changes. I had always defined myself by what I did and how well I did it. Over the next two months, I learned that my heart was a precious gift, and my inner spirit was more important than self-gratification received from high performance. I also absorbed the concept that complete and total healing is a mind, heart, and body experience. Happiness and joy truly come from inside and our eyes and attitudes will reveal this tranquility.

Nursing had opened doors of service and sharing for over four decades, but having cancer, for me, widened those doors with deeper understanding about what total healing is. I have been humbled and strengthened by this chapter in my life, while learning that true healing takes time and a conscious effort. It includes the physical, but also embraces emotional, perceptual, and spiritual elements.

During this past year I have been fortunate to network with many survivors, including previous patients whom I had cared for. A capstone event was the annual Walk for Life this summer, when 150 cancer survivors clasped hands with each other and walked, exposing their personal victories and tears. This was a special occasion for Dave and me. My burden of last year has become my gift for enhancing opportunities to help others who are also coping with cancer.

I am now 62 and have retired from surgical nursing in order to maintain my objectivity. I've chosen a different path of service—in the maternity department caring for new moms and infants. I am also a CPR instructor and teach life-saving techniques to hospital staff and lay people. I'm still jogging and working out three days a week and surrounding myself with good music and positive folks. I laugh a lot and have discovered new avenues of talent in water-color painting and composing poetry.

Anna Quindlen, in her book *a Short Guide to a Happy Life*, states, "Knowledge of our own mortality is the greatest gift God ever gives—because unless you know the clock is ticking, it is so easy to waste our days, our lives."[1] I was chosen to take this journey, and through it I've found peace. I now know how precious life is, and with faith, will live it to its fullest.

---

[1]Quindlen, A *Short Guide to a Happy Life*. 2000. Random House, 64 pages.

CHAPTER 75

WHINING IS ANNOYING

BY BEKA SERDANS

It all began with a stiff neck. My dystonia was first diagnosed by a movement disorder specialist in 1995 although looking back I recall my father remarking on abnormal movements, tremors, and twitches when I was 18 or 19 years old. I've dealt with dystonia for practically half of my life, but was not correctly diagnosed until I was 28 years old. Dystonia is a neurological disorder classified as a movement disorder. It falls within the Parkinson's Disease continuum. Over 350,000 people in North America have the disease, but it often goes undiagnosed because it resembles other movement disorders and many healthcare specialists are unfamiliar with it.

I was born in Germany and lived there for several years, thus am fluent in several languages. At the age of 6, I came to the US, but have spent much time in Europe as well. Most of my education has been in the American education system.

I did what everyone else did in high school. I attended the usual courses in high school in but excelled in the arts and anything that dealt with creativity. I am the oldest of three girls and the only one with dystonia. My two siblings are fit and healthy which at times I envy because I question why I have dystonia and where did I get it from or from whom. Often one struggles with the "why" question. Not knowing why can be torturous to the mind.

At the urging of my father, I entered nursing school and graduated from the University of Rochester with a BSN. I immediately entered critical care nursing after spending only six months working on a cardiac telemetry unit. I like the analytical and technical aspect of critical care nursing. Compassion and empathy evolved and became integral to my practice as I matured professionally.

Symptoms of dystonia slowly developed over time. I noticed abnormal movements of the neck, facial spasms, eyelash spasms, and walking difficulties, along with dystonia of the vocal cords, which gave me a light, breathy voice quality. I diagnosed myself by opening a textbook on neurology and finding a picture of a woman with similar symptoms. The textbook was from the 1950s. Despite visits to several physicians, dystonia was not officially diagnosed until I sought help from the Mount Sinai Movement Disorder Center in New York City. The disorder was suspected in 1994 at the University of Rochester Medical Center, but the complexity of my symptoms baffled the physicians.

I have learned that the more difficult the diagnosis, the less likely one is able to receive an accurate one. Physicians don't think in terms of rarity. I was mislabeled as " stressed-out," "crazy," and I was told "it's all in your head." This was problematic at the time as I was applying to medical school. Once I had an accurate diagnosis, treatment with botulinum toxin (Botox A) began in New York City in 1995. I also entered multiple clinical trials using other drugs.

Initially, I shuttled between Rochester and New York City for treatment, but eventually moved to New York City in 1998. I went to work in critical care at New York Presbyterian Hospital. Currently, I am treated at Columbia's Neurological Institute within their Movement Disorder Division with oral medications and botulinum toxin B (Myobloc). These two toxins temporarily block nerve impulses that induce constant muscle contractions that bring forth the signs of dystonia. The toxin is injected every three months in the most active muscles. Treatment continues as long as one doesn't develop antibodies to the toxin. A cure does not exist. The mechanics of the disease are not yet completely understood, although a gene, the DYT1 gene, has been identified in childhood-onset dystonia.

Working as a nurse with a movement disorder is difficult. I don't think most realize how difficult it is because dystonia is a visible disease. One can hide diabetes, but one can't hide tremors, pain, or abnormal twitching and posturing. With dystonia, one learns to use sensory tricks to hide the disease—body postures that allow one to hide the abnormal movements—but these work for only so long. The actor, Michael J. Fox, was able to hide his Parkinson's Disease for 7 years. Then it interrupted his career. The same applies to me. There is not a day when I do not think about when I no longer will be able to practice critical care nursing. Dystonia grabbed medical school from me, but so far I am able to prevent it from grabbing my career as a nurse. This is something I am constantly afraid of and that I think of on a daily basis.

Many in the intensive care unit do not comprehend dystonia or the amount of effort it takes to hide the abnormal movements or compensate for those movements. I no longer work in the post-anesthesia recovery room because pushing beds is immensely difficult. I end up steering beds with patients into walls, making dents along the hallways.

Walking can be tiresome as it involves spatial orientation. I walk into walls, cut into corners, and cannot always open or crush medications. If I cannot see the task at hand or focus on the task, brain signals are altered and stimulate muscles, inducing the abnormal movements. Using two hands at the same time is difficult. Motor coordination is no longer smooth. Despite these few examples, I rarely ask for help from my colleagues as I have developed a method of nursing care that motivates my patients to help me which helps them in the long run.

Patients constantly ask what is wrong with me. At times I simply say "a stiff neck" or if they question me a bit more I will explain dystonia to them. You might think that I would be more embarrassed more in front of my patients but I am not because they see a quality of nursing not given to them by others. This is not to say that my colleagues provide poor care, but they cannot connect with patients on an emotional level. You cannot learn this unless you have been a patient as well as a nurse.

I am more embarrassed being out on the street because a social stigma exists. I feel safer within the hospital setting as I have taught everyone about dystonia. To a certain degree, however, they know nothing about the disease as they don't live with it on a daily basis. Knowing symptoms is quite different from living with symptoms.

I would not be able to continue working as a critical care nurse (although it is beginning to take a toll) if I did not have the support of everyone who I know at New York Presbyterian—nurses, medical staff, and others. There are high rates of depression, disability, unemployment, and isolation associated with dystonia. The fact that my colleagues are not embarrassed by me and are able to see beyond my movements helps considerably. I consider myself lucky. It means much to me as I initially worked at another hospital for six months where I was ridiculed and laughed at by the nursing staff. The hospital administration didn't want me to participate in a television news story on dystonia because "it would affect their clientele." Now I know what discrimination is. We filmed the program elsewhere.

I still carry my load of patients in the critical care unit. I never take a break, although I do lie down for an hour before the start of the shift. Dystonia eases when you are in the horizontal position. It's the vertical position that brings on problems. No one knows the physics behind this phenomenon. I now ask for help on a more frequent basis as my dystonia has become highly resistant to treatment. I don't see myself as sick, but I do know that my dystonia has progressed over the years. It will most likely end my nursing career in the near future. I am also breaking up my shifts—no longer working 6–12 hour shifts in a row but working 2–3 hours with a rest day in between.

Being a nurse with a disease such as mine has opened up doors that have diminished the impact of loss of previous goals and dreams. I am a writer, patient advocate, and consultant for pharmaceutical companies. I'm the author of two books which describe my daily experiences with dystonia. I have also reentered graduate school, hoping to obtain a Master's degree in nursing.

As a nurse and a patient I realize that multi-disciplinary care is needed for those of us with dystonia. I would sit for hours waiting for my physician to arrive with the toxin. The entire appointment would focus on toxin dosages and rarely would I get an answer to a question or simply be heard as a patient. I would be looked upon as the "TV news girl" or the "nurse" when at times I felt like screaming, "I hate this disease!" I was rarely asked "how are you doing ?" Over time, I began to realize that if this was happening to me, it was also happening to others. By becoming a speaker for a specialized diagnostic testing company, I was able to meet others across the country and collect information about the type of care being provided. Once my audience learned that I was a nurse with dystonia, out came the horror stories which sounded so much like my own. Thus, I knew that optimal dystonia care had never been identified or implemented. That's how I came up with Care4Dystonia, a nonprofit organization focused on setting the pace in areas of public awareness, patient education, and interdisciplinary collaboration.

Over time one learns that quitting is not an option, and whining is annoying. So life goes on—even with dystonia.

CHAPTER 76

IVY

AMY ZLOMEK HEDDEN

I will never forget the first day I laid eyes on Ivy. It was 15 years ago. I was a newly-graduated BSN nurse. I was admitting her to the infectious disease unit where I worked at a children's hospital in Florida. Ivy was about 4 years old. Her scrawny body weighed less than 30 pounds and was short and thin. Her legs were stick-like and she had a protruding abdomen. Her black skin was covered with a dry, raised, cauliflower-like rash that she kept unconsciously scratching at. Her dry, patchy, curly black unkempt hair was wildly springing from her head in every direction. Her chocolate-brown eyes had a wide, sad look to them that seemed older than her actual four years. She had a pouty mouth and her arms were crossed defiantly over her chest.

Ivy's grandmother was with her to provide the necessary admission data. This was the first and last time I saw her grandmother over the many months Ivy spent on our unit. Ivy was HIV-positive. Ivy's mother had been an IV drug user who died recently from AIDS. Ivy's father was not a part of her life. Ivy's maternal grandmother had assumed care of Ivy and her siblings.

I would become Ivy's primary nurse and would care for her over the months to follow. I became not only her nurse, but also her surrogate mother. I gave her medications, bathed her, fed her, combed and braided her hair, rocked her, and read her stories. We played with her many stuffed animals that she received from hospital staff and as donations from various community organizations. She loved to go for rides in a little red wagon. The nurses nicknamed her "Hollywood" because of those wagon rides. She was always dressed to the hilt for those rides. She wore pink sparkly sunglasses shaped like stars, a hot pink visor on her head, and she donned a great big smile. We would have painted her fingernails and toenails too (pink of course). As we drove her through the halls, everyone would tell her how beautiful she was, and she would wave and smile shyly, knowing it was true.

Ivy received many daily medications, most of them were either oral or given intravenously, but one was an injection for her chronic diarrhea. It was ordered twice daily, and was administered twice during my shift. Ivy hated receiving those daily injections and I hated to give them. They were given intramuscularly in her thin thighs, the biggest of all the muscles on her emaciated body. When it was time for her injection I would ensure the help of another nurse or two to hold her still while I gave the injection. As is typical for the growth and development of a preschool child, she would wail, cry, kick, and scream in anticipation of the pain and for several minutes after it's conclusion.

One exceptionally busy day, it was time to administer Ivy's injection and I couldn't find another nurse to help me hold Ivy for her injection. When I entered Ivy's room, a child life therapist, Sunny, was lying in bed with Ivy reading her stories. I warned Ivy that it was time for her injection, and that I still needed to find another nurse to assist me. Sunny offered to hold Ivy for me, and assured me that she had helped the other nurses many times on my days off. I agreed to let Sunny restrain Ivy while I gave the injection. Ivy had already started wailing, crying, kicking and screaming. I closed the door to her room and Sunny put Ivy on her lap and held both legs firmly while I applied gloves and cleansed her left thigh with alcohol. She continued to wail, cry, and scream, but Sunny had her thighs restrained so she could not kick. I gave the injection and as I removed the needle, Sunny released Ivy's legs. Ivy, still having her tantrum, kicked both legs and her left leg caught my right arm and I stuck myself in the middle finger of my left hand with the syringe I had just used to inject Ivy. I screamed in a mixture of surprise and pain. Then reality set in—I had just been stuck with an HIV-positive needle. I ran over to the sink and removed my gloves. I saw blood coming from my middle finger. If I would have had a knife at that moment, I would have cut that finger off without a second thought. Since I didn't, and bandage scissors would never do the job correctly, I turned on the faucet and began to furiously wash and silently cry.

Sunny had been comforting Ivy, who was still crying. Sunny looked up and saw me at the sink with tears running down my face. She asked me what had happened. I numbly told her I had stuck myself with Ivy's syringe. Sunny gently placed Ivy back in her bed and ran to call the infectious disease nurse. I just stood quietly at the sink looking at my bleeding finger under the water still coming from the faucet.

Jan, the infectious disease nurse, arrived. She gently took me by the arm and led me from Ivy's room. Jan questioned me about the incident. She was stern, matter-of-fact, and offered me no sympathy or emotional support. She asked whether I was wearing gloves, if the child had been adequately restrained, and if I used the proper technique to administer the medication. I felt like a criminal. She handed me a form to fill out and asked me to submit it at the end of my shift. She told me that she would arrange to have a blood specimen taken to determine my current HIV status, and then routine successive specimens would be drawn to watch for any changes.

Something inside me snapped. I told Jan that it was now the end of my shift. She looked at me surprised, and told me that I could not leave immediately, because there was no one to replace me. I informed Jan that she had better find someone quickly, because I was in no state of mind to continue my shift and provide care to my patients. I told her I had been married less than one year, and had a husband at home who would have no one to replace me either if I died from AIDS.

I left the floor and went to the lab to have my baseline HIV status drawn. My eyes were red and puffy. My face was flushed. The receptionist noticed my sadness and asked me what was wrong. I calmly stated I had just been stuck by a needle from a small child with AIDS. She patted my arm and told me that God gave special protection to nurses who cared for children with AIDS, and assured me I'd be ok.

Somehow I made it to my car. I was sad, angry, and ready to never go back to nursing again. I drove directly to my church. I said a prayer, asking for forgiveness for all the wrongs I'd committed in my life and asking for mercy. I wanted to raise children with my husband and live to see them grow old. I wanted to continue to care for all the sick children on my unit at the hospital, but I didn't want to jeopardize my own health in the process.

When I arrived at home, I called my husband who came home and held me while I cried. I told him he would need to wear condoms from now on when we had sex to reduce his risk of contracting HIV, in the event I became HIV positive. I told him I would understand if he didn't want to kiss me or have sex with me at all anymore. My husband said to me, "If you get HIV and die, I'll want to die to. We are not living our lives any differently than we have in the past."

I called in sick to work the next two days as I contemplated my career and my fate. My husband sent me flowers with encouraging notes. I began to feel less sorry for myself and had faith that perhaps God did give special protection to nurses. I began to miss my colleagues and my patients.

I returned to nursing and to my position caring for children on the infectious disease unit. Psychologically, I wasn't able to care for Ivy immediately after I returned. After a few weeks I was able to care for her again, but could never bring myself to again administer her injections.

Ivy died about one year later from complications related to AIDS. In the final days of her life the nurses on our unit took turns staying around the clock at her bedside so she would not have to die alone. After her death, each nurse who was emotionally involved with her kept one of her stuffed animals.

It's been fifteen years since I first cared for Ivy. I live in California now, have two children, and am still married to my wonderful husband. Ivy's gray bunny with the flowered dress is in my hope chest. When I see it, I am reminded of a little girl who was born with an incurable illness. I hope that she is at peace and in heaven, riding around in a little red wagon, wearing sparkly star-shaped sunglasses, a hot pink visor, with pink-painted fingernails and toenails, wearing a great big smile. I also remember that God does give special protection to nurses.

CHAPTER 77

THE SPOILS OF WAR

BY STEVEN L. BROWN

Somewhere in Iraq, there is a man. This man is a victim of war, shot by his fellow countrymen after being suspected of aiding an invading force. Born and raised in Iraq, he lived under a single man's rule for the majority of his life.

During his life, our man was told that Americans were evil. The Infidels, as Americans were called in the schools, would do terrible things to the people of his nation if they succeeded in their invasion. Naturally, as a patriotic father and a family man, he carried these lessons forward and relayed stories of these horrific people to his countrymen. This is what is taught in Iraqi schools, in Iraqi families, and in every aspect of Iraqi lives.

Our man, however, got a first-hand look at The Infidels after being taken to a U.S. Navy fleet hospital in southern Iraq. He had been shot in the chest and needed emergent surgical treatment in order to survive. He was brought to the U.S. Navy's Fleet Hospital 3 for medical treatment afforded to him as part of the Geneva Convention. After his surgery, he was admitted to the intensive care unit for recovery and critical care monitoring. Our man recovered quickly from his surgical procedure, and was awaiting transport to another facility for follow-up care.

After several days, and many hours of seeing my colleagues and I care for his fellow countrymen in the same manner as we cared for our own beloved American fighting men and women, he called me to his bedside. As I approached, I noticed tears in his eyes. I came to him and inquired what was the matter. He simply looked at me and began to weep. His heart was breaking, but I didn't know why. Regaining his composure, he began to speak. He whispered that after seeing the nursing care he and his fellow countrymen had been receiving he had been filled with guilt and remorse.

"The Chicken Farmer," as he was affectionately known (because of his vocation), went on to explain that he had ascribed to his country's notions regarding the United States, otherwise known to him as The Evil Empire. He spoke of lectures to his children and his persistent assurance that his family felt the same hate toward Americans as the rest of his countrymen did. "How can I face my children now," he said, "after everything that has happened?" He had come to the realization through the caring and compassion shown to him and the rest of the patients at FH-3, that The Infidels weren't all that bad. In fact, they were actually a good people, a people who cared for others and showed respect, dignity, and compassion for all that entered its compound regardless of nationality or activity prior to arriving. As his tears welled up again, he returned to thoughts of his children and the lessons he had taught them in his own home. He replayed them in his mind, only to realize the harm he had done in perpetuating his country's mindset.

I was speechless. Here I was, a Navy Nurse Corps Officer in a war zone, somewhere in the desert of southern Iraq, caring for a citizen of a country we had invaded. I was watching "The Chicken Farmer" come to a new realization, after seeing the care he and others received. I stood in silence and offered my hand in understanding. He readily took it and squeezed tightly as he continued to cry.

The rest of his stay at the fleet hospital was fun to watch for the staff. He quickly became an ambassador for the United States within the ICU. He spoke his native Arabic to fellow patients, explaining where they were, and that they too would be receiving the same quality care he had. He was trying to convey his new found reality to others in the unit, allaying fears and providing some comfort of his own. Many were relieved to see a fellow countryman telling them these things.

Somewhere in Iraq, there is a man—a man changed by the care he received from nurses at an American Navy fleet hospital. These are the spoils of war.

Chapter 78

The Patient I Hated

By Amy Blanchard

All names in the following story have been changed. This is written from my perspective as a nurse and is in no way a reflection of the views of the United States Army. All thoughts and feelings are purely a reflection of my experience. I would like to dedicate this to Sallman and all of our soldiers continuing to fight for Iraq's freedom.

His name was Enemy Prisoner of War (EPW) 270. He was a patient of mine on the night shift in Iraq. Actually, his name was Sallman, but that didn't matter to me. To me he was nothing more than EPW 270. He was the abscess in the neck, post grenade fragment in Bed 14. He was the 270th enemy soldier wounded while he was attempting to kill U.S. forces. He was the 270th enemy soldier that a US pilot risked his own life for, by flying him to our hospital so that we could save him. He was the 270th EPW keeping me thousands of miles away from my family in the middle of the desert of Iraq.

I hated him because I had sat in trenches while scuds flew over my head. I hated him because I had been drinking hot water and sleeping in 130 degree tents for four months. I hated him because I had been blinded by sandstorms so fierce that the skies turned red. I hated him because even when I did get to shower my body and my clothes were still coated with dirt and sand. I hated EPW 270. I hated him! I hated him when I slept, and I hated him when I was awake. Every night I hated him more and more. I hated him so much that sometimes I couldn't breathe. I hated him so much that tears stung my eyes whenever I heard him call out to me for help. I hated to look at his pale and gaunt face. I hated to smell him and the purulent, foul pus draining out from his neck. I hated to touch his clammy, cold flesh. I hated him in every possible way and I hated being his nurse. I hated him!

Hating him made me miserable. I couldn't stop hating him though. I didn't *want* to stop hating him. I thought that if somehow I hated him enough he would disappear and that I wouldn't have to be his nurse anymore. He never disappeared. Each night when I came into work he was there in Bed 14 waiting for me—waiting for his dressing changes, his tube feeds, his pain medication, his urine to be dumped, his JP drains to be emptied, his antibiotics to be hung, his labs to be drawn. And I was there, every night, his nurse, hating every minute of every night with EPW 270.

It was 02:42 on a Wednesday morning. I remember glancing at my watch when over the radio I heard "Attention on the net, attention on the net, one US emergent litter gun shot wound to the right femur en route." Seconds later I heard the sixth Blackhawk medivac helicopter of the night land outside on our landing pad. EPW 270 hadn't been sleeping at all that night. He was demanding and cranky, spilling urine on the floor, spitting on his sheets, constantly calling "Sister! Sister!" to tell me "La Nam! La Nam! (No sleep! No sleep!). I decided a sleeping pill was in order and headed straight to the place I knew I would find a doctor awake at this time of night—the emergency room.

I ducked in, coughing on the dust and sand I was kicking up along my way. I looked up from writing a note on the chart when I reached the ER. Nothing I had seen yet in the war compared to what I saw then. I had seen missing legs, missing arms, missing faces. I had seen more blood than a thousand cheap horror films. I had seen starving and diseased children. But this time, what I saw drove a knife of sadness and grief right into my heart.

A soldier lay on a litter in front of me. His body was a dusky purple. His face was turned away from me, but I could tell that the naked soldier lying there in front of me was lifeless. There were no major wounds that I saw, no massive amounts of blood. No drama of the nurses trying to save his life. The soldier had bled so much on his way to the hospital that he didn't have much blood left to bleed by the time he got there. He was the gunshot wound to the femur that had been called in over the radio. His left arm suddenly flopped off of the litter and dangled at his side. A bright gleam drew my eyes to his hand. It was a wedding ring. I wanted to crumple to the floor and sob. The reality of the war I was in suddenly slapped me right across the face. I had images of a wife and children at home receiving the devastating news that their husband and father were dead, their lives to never be the same again.

I spun around on my heels and stomped back to the EPW ward, without ever getting an order for EPW 270. As far as I was concerned, I didn't care if he ever slept again. I wanted him to suffer like the family of that soldier was going to suffer. I walked right up to 270 and told him to 'be quiet' in Arabic and to just go to sleep because he would be getting no sleeping medication. I couldn't hold back the tears that sprung up in my eyes and started to run down my cheeks. I stared at him in defiance, before turning and storming off into the back room where I attempted to choke back my tears so the other prisoners wouldn't think I was losing control. Moments later, my good friend, Nabil, who interpreted for our hospital, came into the back of the tent and placed his hands on my shoulders.

"Amy," he said, "Sallman asked me why you hate him."

"Who is Sallman?" I asked Nabil, wiping my nose with a paper towel.

"You know, 270," said Nabil. In a gentle and quiet voice Nabil said, "Come here, I want you to speak with him."

Before I could say no, Nabil grabbed my hand and pulled me over to 270's bed. 270 was crying. His face was in his hands and he was crying hard. He looked up when he felt me standing next to him with Nabil. His face was twisted and contorted with emotion. He looked suddenly very vulnerable to me. What proceeded was a passionate conversation between an angry, sad American nurse and an angry, sad Iraqi man. As Nabil interpreted I learned that 270 had never raised a violent hand against the Americans. It was his brother who had thrown a grenade at U.S. troops. Sallman was at his side, torn between love for his brother and hate for Saddam Hussein's regime. Sallman was injured when one of the grenades his brother threw detonated too close and sent shrapnel flying into his neck. He was arrested because he was in the wrong place at the wrong time. Sallman had three babies and he was very worried about them. His wife had no money to feed or care for them. He didn't know where they were or if they were dead or alive. As I listened to Sallman's story I realized it wasn't Sallman that I hated. I hated the war and all the suffering it caused on both sides. I hated being away from my family. I hated seeing my fellow Americans get killed and then have to turn around and nurse those that had killed them. I hated the regime that caused the war and caused the suffering of innocent people that I had seen.

I realized that I had misdirected that hate onto Sallman. Sallman was no longer EPW 270. I now saw him as Sallman. Sallman was a husband and father. He was a sibling who had lost his brother. He was a human being, not a number. He wasn't a pharyngeal abscess anymore. I truly saw him as my patient for the first time. My patient had a heart, a mind, and a soul, just like mine.

By the night's end, I had taken Sallman's hand in mine in friendship and peace. Over the next several weeks, Sallman and I became friends. He taught me how to count to ten in Arabic and helped me greatly improve the Arabic I spoke. I taught him card tricks. He "oohed" and "ahhed" over care packages I received from home. We watched DVDs together and listened to music. We shared many laughs. I comforted him when he was in pain and he'd pat me on the arm when I was lonesome for home. There we were, two people who couldn't have less in common, who somehow managed to break through language and cultural barriers and the tragedies of war to become friends.

Sallman saved me. He saved me from losing sight of why I became a nurse. He reminded me that it's not medicine and surgery and dressing changes that heal patients. These things serve only to treat patients. Instead it's compassion and a tender heart and tender hand that heal. A nurse isn't a nurse unless she or he maintains that tenderness and compassion. Sallman also taught me that our patients can heal us as much as we can heal them. I helped Sallman heal his wounds, and he helped me heal my hate.

CHAPTER 79

A FAMILY AFFAIR

BY ELIZABETH SAMER

I was working in the emergency department of my local medical center. It was the twelfth hour of my thirteen-hour shift. Like all of us, I was looking forward to the arrival of the next shift. Then a paramedic called, specifically requesting to speak with me. The paramedics were on a call for an 80-year-old man with a history of high blood pressure. He had been in his normal state of health when he had a sudden onset of speech disturbance and weakness on his left side. The symptoms began one hour prior to the arrival of the paramedics.

The paramedic on duty called me to ask if my son, John, was still on duty for the medical transport service that he worked for on the weekends. The paramedic and his partner faced a problem, as transportation of patients to the hospital in our town is usually accomplished through volunteer squads and the fire rescue team. The paramedic quickly explained that the patient was a prime candidate for the use of TPA (tissue plaminogen activator) or the "clot buster"—a drug used to treat stroke victims. He gave me a short report of the patient's symptoms, which strongly suggested a stroke in evolution. He told me that the patient had no contraindications for the use of TPA, such as trauma or a history of bleeding disorders. This patient was well within the three-hour window of opportunity for the use of the clot-busting drug. Treatment after this three hour window is usually unsuccessful in eliminating or minimizing the affects of the cerebral vascular accident (CVA) or stroke and the risk or bleeding usually outweighs the benefit.

The paramedics were unable to get a transport team together from the town they were in. They had tried all the recourses available to them and were thinking outside of the box. Could I get hold of my son? I said, "Hold on." I tried my son on his cell phone. He and his crew were heading back to base as their shift was almost over. Acting as a go-between, I gave my son the address for the paramedic call. We directed the transport team, with their lights on and sirens wailing, to the address. They were able to bring the acutely ill patient into the medical facility well within the time frame for the use of life-saving drug therapy.

I did not stay to witness the effects of therapy. It had been a very long thirteen-hour shift and I needed to give report and finalize the medical records of patients already in my care. I have long since come to terms with the fact that the outcome for some patients lies in powers outside of our control. We had acted as a team to ensure safe and timely delivery of emergency care, and we had been creative in problem-solving to ensure the best medical care for this patient. Sometimes that is enough.

CHAPTER 80

FROM CLASSROOM TO BEDSIDE

BY ARLENE M. CLARKE-COUGHLIN

The conference before a day in the hospital can teach students lifelong lessons. The conference is an opportunity for each student to present their patient's case and explore their data. I have found this period of time a valuable learning tool for my students. As an instructor, I often change the way the conference is handled. While it is important for the instructor to determine that all of the students are prepared for their assignment, it's also a great opportunity to role play and allow the students to practice how they might interact in a given situation.

One day I had a group of students preparing to care for their patients in the intensive care setting. Instead of delving into pathophysiology and pharmacology I decided to role play with several students. I had two students caring for a 32-year-old comatose woman who was critically ill and was preparing to go to the operating room for a tracheostomy. Another set of two students were caring for an 82-year-old comatose man. This man was in multi system organ failure. I could see that these students had reams of paper to support the clinical steps they wanted to take, but I felt that the psychological aspects of critical illness were also pertinent issues. Therefore I changed the tenor of the conference and role played with each group.

Case 1: Maria was a 32-year-old Hispanic female. She was suffering from complications following stomach surgery. She was in shock, on a ventilator, and in a coma. Maria was the mother of a 12-year-old girl and her husband had just signed permission for this procedure the night before. The two students who were caring for Maria presented an overview of her illness. I told the students that I would be playing the role of Maria's husband.

I looked at the students and said in a distraught and panicked manor, "Nurses, my wife Maria—is she going to die? Please help me. What is going to happen to her?" The students looked stunned, almost like deer paralyzed in the headlights of a car. They responded, "Oh, let me get your nurse." I told the students that Maria's' nurse was on break and they had to interact with Maria's husband. The two students were befuddled and struggled to find something to say. I persisted in my distraught manor pleading, "Is Maria going to die?" Slowly the students began to relax and answer the questions that I posed to them in a caring and compassionate manner. I took this opportunity to stress to the group the importance of communication techniques—warmth of compassion and the therapeutic use of touch. I also stressed to the group that the family is their patient, too. Being a good nurse is to incorporate the family into the plan of care for the person receiving treatment.

Case 2: The second set of students was caring for an 82-year-old man who had multiple-system failure and was in the process of dying. Earlier in the morning I had helped the students with their morning assessments and had observed Mr. Davis. He had a bad night. He was unshaven, sweating, and had spattered blood on his face and hair. His family (five daughters and a wife), had been at his bedside constantly, but took a few hours to freshen up and have a needed cup of coffee.

At the conference I asked the students what this patients priority need was. The ten students in the conference yelled in unison "Airway, breathing, and circulation!" I responded "No," and the ten students looked at me with disbelief. We then discussed family, critical illness, and death. I discussed with them my personal philosophy of nursing and went on to say that you should treat every patient the way that you would want your mother or father cared for. I explained that this man was dying and that no nursing or medical intervention was going to change the outcome. The students all agreed that his priority was comfort. His physical appearance was not very comforting right now. They wanted to bathe him, shave him and make him look better for his family. We went on to talk about how we could meet the psychological needs of his wife and daughters. We role played on how they, as his nurses, could respond to the family by offering compassion and warmth during this time.

The conference was over, and I told the students that were caring for Mr. Davis that I would help them with his hygiene and comfort needs. At the nurses station we were discussing what we needed to do for him. From the corner of my eye I noticed the two students who were working with Maria. Running down the hall was Maria's husband. He was crying out "Madre Dios! My Maria, is she going to die?"

I watched as the husband entered into Maria's room. The two students were with him since Maria's primary nurse was at coffee. I tried to get the students' attention, but watched with pride as they spoke with the husband calmly. One student put her arm around his shoulder and continued to talk with him. I got her attention and mouthed to her across the nurse's station, "Do you need me?" The student's eyes and face said it all. She waved me away with her hand and closed the door.

In the meantime, I helped the other two students with Mr. Davis. We washed and shaved him, making him look more comfortable. The cardiac monitor showed a very slow heart rate of 20 beats per minute. Mr. Davis had a do not resuscitate order. Just then, the wife and daughters returned. They looked at Mr. Davis and gulped. Tears rolled down their faces and the wife said, "God bless you, John looks so well cared for." One of the students then brought up a chair and lowered the side rail by John's head. She put the chair next to the patient and offered the chair to his wife. His wife sat down next to him and then the student invited her to kiss his face. The wife asked, "Is John dying?" I looked at the student and she replied, "His body is losing the fight. Here, come and be with him." The second student said, "Mrs. Davis, would you like a priest?" The priest came instantly. John passed away in the warmth and comfort of his family. They were all very grateful and embraced the students when they left.

A good nurse is not just someone who knows pathophysiology and pharmacology. A good nurse also knows how to provide compassion and warmth to their patients. I consider myself very lucky. I have the opportunity to help mold future nurses and to stress to them what it means to be a good nurse.

CHAPTER 81

9-11-01

BY BONNIE WHAITE

September 11, 2001 is a day of sorrow, permanently etched in most American's hearts and minds. As with the day that John F. Kennedy was assassinated, my activities from that day will be forever crystal clear in my memory. What was different for me during this more recent tragic day was that I viewed the events from a nursing perspective. This day in history taught me much about nursing and the people of our profession.

The early part of this Tuesday morning started out in the usual way. I was up and out the door by 6:00 am to go to my clinical site at the local hospital. This was the first day of a 14-week pediatric clinical experience for my ten nursing students. Most had never been on a pediatric unit before. I had planned to start the day with a short tour of the facility and an orientation to pediatric procedures and policies. After this, each student would be assigned a patient and family for whom they would provide care.

The first day on a pediatric rotation often causes students much anxiety. Most of their prior experiences have been with adults. Infants and small children are different and a little foreign. Students also have to adjust to a new instructor, a new location, different equipment, and new nursing staff. My ten fourth-semester BSN students were no different. I could sense their stress immediately.

Our short orientation went well and everyone seemed a little more relaxed about this first day on pediatrics. The students received their patient assignments and went off to meet the families, do assessments, and start morning care. A short time later, a student, looking very anxious, came to me saying that her assigned family had said that there was a TV news bulletin of a plane crash in New York City. The plane had hit the World Trade Center. My immediate response was to ask, "Are you sure? This doesn't seem possible, but talk to your family and keep them and yourself calm." Soon, another concerned student found me and said that she had seen the same news flash on the television in her patient's room. Slowly, all of us on pediatrics that day—patients, families, instructor, students, nurses, residents, and physicians—began to realize that something horrific was happening in our country.

All televisions and radios were turned on and we tried to catch whatever reports were available. The media began giving us a barrage of information about New York City, the World Trade Center, Washington D.C., and Pennsylvania. There were terrible images of death and destruction that shocked us. Even though we were far away from these places, our hearts were full of fear, shock, sadness, and dismay. One couldn't help but think, 'would we be next?'

My students were quiet and afraid. I gathered all ten together and we discussed what they were feeling and how best to proceed with the day. My own emotions were in turmoil and I initially thought to send them home since this was only their first day. As we talked among ourselves these wonderful students decided that they would stay the rest of the clinical day. They felt that they could be of help to the patients, their families, and the nursing staff on this terrible day. They would continue to work and try to be a calm resource in a time of chaos. I saw courage in my students at this moment. I gave them the option to leave and be with their own families, but they choose to stay and help their patients in whatever way possible. I was touched by their thoughtfulness and caring spirits.

The pediatric staff nurses were also doing their best to keep patients and families calm and to provide the nursing care that was required. Many of these nurses had personal connections to family and friends in New York City or Washington D.C. The assistant nurse manager's sister, brother-in-law, and niece were stationed at a military base in Washington D.C. She was very concerned for their safety. One of my own student's parents live and work in New York City. He, too, was fearful for their safety. For part of this awful day neither of these people had any information as to the safety of their loved ones, yet they maintained their composure. The assistant nurse manager and my student both provided their patients with physical, emotional, and spiritual nursing care that is required of our calling as nurses no matter how we are feeling.

As the day passed and we knew the truth about the terrorist acts in New York City, Pennsylvania, and Washington D.C., all of us experienced a deep sense of sadness and loss. There was sadness for the thousands who had perished and grief for the families left behind. There was also a sense of loss for the destruction of property, but even more distinct was the loss of feeling safe and secure in our country.

I was glad when the time came to leave the hospital and to go home to my own family. Yet I was also proud of what the nursing staff and my students had accomplished during this day of crisis and fear. Watching and being a part of this nursing experience taught me much about what makes nurses (and student nurses) so unique and special. I saw nurses who had their own deep feelings of sorrow and anxiety continue to provide compassionate nursing care to sick patients and families who were greatly distressed by these acts of violence. I observed the nurses and student nurses who might have wanted to put their own needs first, provide a calm, caring environment for sick children and their families.

I felt a deep sense of pride for my own ten students who made the decision, on their first day of a new clinical experience, to remain working and learning in extremely difficult circumstances. I saw in these students the "art of nursing" which includes compassion, caring, and commitment. This group of ten students has since graduated. I am confident that they are practicing nursing with compassion and expertise. They have no doubt become RNs who are a valued asset to our profession.

During this day I saw what makes nurses so special in providing healthcare to others. Our uniqueness was visibly expressed on this pediatric unit September 11, 2001. Nurses have heart and at the same time are strong and resilient. This experience, terrible as it was, reminds me of how proud I am to be a nurse and a part of the nursing profession.

CHAPTER 82

THE NEW MANAGER

BY JANICE KAY HIBLER FREEMAN

In 1988 the head nurse position on 9 Purple, an oncology nursing unit where I worked as a charge nurse, became available. I recall the struggle of deciding whether or not to make a career move and pursue the position. First of all, I had little management experience, and secondly, our nursing unit had a negative and unpopular reputation within the organization. Could I manage a team with such a reputation, negative attitudes, competition among team members, personal clashes, and dissatisfied patients and physicians? Although I did not know the answer, I did know that our patients needed quality nursing care and that the nursing team was capable of providing just that.

Early in the day, a co-worker who had a great deal of faith in me, asked if I had made the decision. She tried to offer her reassurance by telling me, "Don't worry, you can do it!" I knew I could give quality nursing care as an individual, but then I wondered if I could provide even more care through others.

The nursing director visited our unit, and asked if I had given consideration to apply. Still waning, I remembered the encouragement of my co-worker. Then, with determination to help the patients receive quality nursing care and improve the unit's reputation, I grabbed a paper towel from the nearby dispenser and wrote a quick note indicating my intent to apply for the head nurse position. In my heart I knew this was the right decision, but in my mind, I thought I was experiencing a moment of temporary insanity. Somewhat surprised by my choice in stationary, the nursing director accepted the paper-towel note, and several weeks later I accepted the job as the new head nurse.

Upon accepting the head nurse position, I decided upon two goals. The first goal was to take care of the people who were ill and secondly take care of the people who are providing the care to those that are ill. I visualized our unit functioning as an old junky car. Various parts were detached, torn, mangled, or missing. Our car was stationary, unable to move. I recognized what parts needed to come together, which needed replacing or rebuilding. I also visualized how the nursing unit, or car, would appear when all the parts were smoothly working together and able to move forward. Several basic components needed to be in place before any other building could occur and before we could move forward. One of the basic components that did exist was a clinical expert available to the nursing staff. Our unit was very fortunate to have a Clinical Nurse Specialist who provided clinical direction, guidance, and education for each level of nursing personnel. In addition, our unit received leadership support from our nursing director. The individuals working on this hospital floor comprised the last component. Each individual had their own personality, strengths, weaknesses, hidden agendas, and skills. Often this individuality created conflict and unpleasant emotions. There were hurt feelings, grudges, silence, and competition among the individuals. I wondered how such a group could participate toward one goal.

As I tried to sort out the issues and problems with the staff, facing angry patients, family, staff, and doctors became a daily routine. Crying alone in my office became a routine, too. Nursing staff that I thought were supportive of me, now were talking unfavorably about my efforts. We had limited nursing resources to provide care to such a great number of ill patients. Nursing staff from other areas in the hospital did not want to work with us because our unit was deemed unfriendly, and had "attitude". One of the observant patients approached me to share her advice. She encouraged me not to give up on my vision and not to let the turkeys in the staff get me down. I realized that I was letting the turkeys get me down. It was time to bring the goal and the visualization to the team.

There were discussions among the staff about the good points and the bad points both with individuals and with the team, and how these points impacted the quality of care. In addition, meetings were held with individuals to identify what their goals and visions included. Needs of the individual as well as those of the team were important and had to be addressed. The team was challenged to make a decision about the delivery of patient care both now and in the future. Soon, ideas were created and implemented. The nursing team was starting to work together and take charge of their destiny.

Our unit did not change overnight. Gradually, there were fewer angry patients, family, nursing staff, and doctors. Amazingly, patients requested placement on our hospital floor, and doctors rewarded the nursing staff with compliments and goodies. Other nurses asked to work on our unit, and student nurses wanted to join our team. Some of the most challenging drug regimes, which required coordination of care and clinical nursing knowledge, were assigned to our unit. We received many cards and letters from patients who expressed gratitude for the compassionate, friendly, and high-quality nursing care they received while on our hospital floor. The teamwork and professionalism were often mentioned in these letters. Nursing staff from other units sent cards and letters, too, recognizing the team's cohesiveness, cooperation, and friendliness. Several nurses said that they looked forward to working with us in the future, not so much for the extra pay, but to have the opportunity to work with such a supportive team. Our nursing leaders acknowledged our outstanding caregivers and our team with commendations. Individual team members pursued higher education and returned to work with the same team as advanced practice nurses. We recognized that a good working atmosphere contributes to good patient outcomes. As a team, we were proud of and amazed by our accomplishments.

Reflecting on my experience as a new head nurse, I realized that everyone on a nursing team contributes in his or her own way. Some participate on the front line, others participate behind the scenes, and others pave the way for good things to happen. The nursing staff learned that it is okay to be both an individual and part of a team. Thank you to each individual who contributed to the high-quality patient care that we now deliver to our patients while they stay on our hospital unit—the unit called 9 Purple, alias 8 LP. Thank you to the patient who was willing to share her observations and advice on what it takes to be a manager.

CHAPTER 83

SNAPSHOTS

BY MARY KATE DILTS SKAGGS

Nephrology nursing is the technical term for caring for patients who have kidney disease, some of whom need kidney dialysis. Nephrology nursing will always be special for me because of the relationship one develops with patients and their families due to the chronic nature of kidney failure.

In 1984, I became a staff nurse in a dialysis unit. The first day I reported to work was late in October and I was told to "dress up" for work. I wore pink tights with a navy blue flowered dress, a big bow tied in my hair, and I carried a stuffed animal. I guess I should have known that I was headed for an exciting career at that point in time.

Over the years, our dialysis unit had a Hawaiian Luau, Halloween parties, and a Christmas party. I can remember a Christmas party when my younger brother, who was in college, came to call bingo during one of the dialysis treatment sessions. When all of the patients' dialysis treatments were started, the nurses had all gotten together and made stockings for the patients. Many of our patients were poor and we realized that some of them might not receive any Christmas gifts except what the nursing staff brought for them.

We played bingo often and a lot of the staff donated prizes. I didn't realize it at the time, but one of the nurses had written a bingo number on a Band-Aid and slipped it to my brother who was calling bingo. The staff rigged the bingo night so that all the patients won at least one game. The staff called our bingo games "dirty bingo," and I, as the nurse manager at this time, was unaware of what the staff had orchestrated. Another fond memory is that some of my patients and their families attended my wedding reception. I often joke that my patients saw me grow up as a staff nurse, get engaged, get married, get pregnant, and change jobs to become a manager.

Another Halloween, I can remember looking out the window and watching Elmer, who was in a wheelchair, being pushed by his son Don across the parking lot. Not only was the staff dressing up in costumes, we had told the patients that they could dress up. To my delight, Elmer had decided that he would wear his overalls and plaid shirt, like he did on many occasions, but he had a red bandana that he put across his face when he came through the doors of the dialysis unit, like he was a bandit. Years later when Elmer died, I remember speaking with Elmer's family at the funeral home. They told me how much he looked forward to coming to dialysis that day because the staff and the patients were wearing costumes. These little things that we have done have made a difference to our patients and their families.

Another fond memory I have is the 50th anniversary party that the nursing staff put together. There was a dialysis patient named Forrest who had a wife named Marie. They never had any children. Forrest was on dialysis and they had been married for 50 years. The nursing staff got together, had an anniversary cake baked, and we had a little party for them in the dialysis unit and served cake to all the patients, families, and staff.

Another warm memory I have as a nephrology nurse who spent 12 years working in dialysis is that I had a brother who had a part-time job working at the dialysis unit taking inventory of supplies. As my career changed, I became a regional administrator and was managing three dialysis units in Ohio and Kentucky. I received a phone call one day and one of the nurses said, "Could we train James to be a dialysis technician?" I said, "Well, I guess you should talk to James." That was never my intention. He just did the inventory and helped with ordering, but if the nurses and James were interested, I would give them my blessing.

Over the course of time the nurses did train James. He became a dialysis technician. He developed a wonderful rapport with patients, and six years later James graduated with an associates degree in nursing. Today James is a director of nursing of three units in Ohio. It is almost as if he has followed in his sister's footsteps. One of my proudest moments was being at his nursing school pinning and college graduation, knowing that sometimes we are not aware that we are role models and that we have a great influence on other people in our lives.

CHAPTER 84

OCCUPATIONAL HEALTH NURSING

BY ANNMARIE CENTRONE-CEFOLI

Occupational health nursing is a specialty practice wherein one takes care of employees in the workplace. One wears many hats from healthcare provider, to health educator, to manager, to promoter of safety programs, to coordinator of disability and worker's compensation management.

No two days are the same. We may respond to an epileptic seizure—we remove the person from her work area and bring her to the health unit, until she recovers. We are sometimes called because someone has collapsed and has had a heart attack. Mundane things, like monitoring an employee's blood pressure, sugar level for a diabetic, weight or cholesterol are opportunities to teach and to support an employee's attempts to improve their health. We really celebrate when someone quits smoking or loses the weight they need to.

One story that fills me with pride is about Amy, who had a pregnancy-related problem. She wanted to be a mother badly, but her pregnancy was very high-risk. She received permission to get a medication that she needed that is administered by an injection at work. She came to the health unit regularly to get the injection. While the medication was needed to sustain the pregnancy, one of the scary possible side effects was fetal abnormality. What a joy when she gave birth to a health baby girl. I felt so much a part of this miraculous event!

Worker's compensation management is extremely important in terms of cost containment and accident prevention. This is an area where a nurse can have a real impact on a company's bottom line. Immediate onsite treatment of health problems, reporting and referring to reputable healthcare facilities, correction of workplace hazards, and accident prevention training are key aspects of an occupational health nurse's job. Dealing with employees, their families, healthcare providers, insurance companies, and the manager on the job can be time consuming and tedious, but these are rewarding tasks when the employee and the workplace emerge in a better condition than before.

CHAPTER 85

ALL IN A DAY'S WORK

By JoAnn Brakora Bugbee

Today is the Education Fair, 7:00 am–5:00 pm; the day dawns bright and clear.

A TV and its VCR are not in place for a learning activity.

Not all refreshments arrived as scheduled.

An unscheduled person arrives on the scene, but he is so conscientious. Make the necessary paperwork.

An important piece of resuscitation equipment is missing.

A resuscitation instructor calls and says he is 'unable' to come, but then a scheduled substitute shows up! Whew!

A live presenter is nowhere to be found, and it's five minutes after the scheduled start of the presentation! No substitutes are available, and no learning materials exist for two of the learning activities. A second TV and VCR suddenly aren't there. Announce that the learning activity is temporarily postponed to a potentially hostile crowd and escape unscathed. What to do next?

It's only shortly after 8:00 am.

Unable to attend the pre-arranged teleconference off site due to all of above. (Small wonder.)

Retrieve missing piece of resuscitation equipment.

Ransack a colleague's office, with security escort just to be safe, and voila! Find not one, but two videos to choose from, a poster, and learning materials for the missing activity. Try previewing the videos on the spot, but that TV and VCR do not work!

A TV and VCR arrive at the learning site, but emits very loud popping sounds and starts to smoke! An audio-visual man promptly removes the offensive equipment before it can set off the smoke detector. (Wouldn't that be fun!) Oh well, there is a back up TV (lucky me) and he'll check on the other VCR that won't play.

The backup TV and VCR aren't working either. (Why do I get the feeling this isn't my day?) But, the third one "just needed to be reprogrammed; all the channels had been deleted." (And they say there's no such thing as gremlins!)

Pick up camera from one of the nursing units and take a few pictures for our accreditation project. (That went smoothly; something must be wrong here!)

Make video selection for the temporarily postponed program. Hope they like it!

Make extra handouts and reference materials for the missing speaker presentation. (There, that should still meet all the learning objectives.)

A fire alarm sounds on one of the units!

Time for the temporarily postponed program, and staff ask for extra credit for the unauthorized hands-on training they've just participated in. Imagine that!

Return camera to unit and arrange to pick up supply of popcorn. Arrive at Canteen. "We're so sorry. We forgot to tell you the popcorn machine is broken! But a new one is on order. And, we're out of chips which would make a good substitute, right?" That's OK. There must just be something about today.

Eat lunch. Grateful for small things today.

Missed a scheduled afternoon meeting.

Education materials finally get taken down and packed up for the day, after a false start.

Ready to go home, and guess what! The toilet overflowed!

CHAPTER 86

PARISH NURSING

BY CARYL A. PRATI

I am a parish nurse at St. Andrew Catholic Church in Moore, Oklahoma. This position developed as a direct result of the May 3, 1999 tornado that devastated southern Oklahoma. I had just relocated to Oklahoma City in March to be with my husband who had taken a new job there. We had decided to register as members at St. Andrew. St. Andrew had over 100 families who suffered complete or minor damage to their homes. I wanted to help, but I was very new to the area. Within a couple of weeks, Catholic Charities, an agency offering community relief, asked me to become a liaison with our parish to help the families that had been so devastated. I volunteered in this capacity for six months.

Catholic Charities had actively funded the first full-time parish nurse position in Oklahoma City two years prior to this May 3rd event. In November of 1999 Catholic Charities offered to partially fund a three-year pilot parish nurse position at St. Andrew because it recognized that there would be long-term needs. My pastor, Father Jack, eagerly supported this offer and asked me to consider it. I did not know what parish nursing entailed, but Catholic Charities had agreed to act as a co-sponsor with St. Anthony Hospital to bring the first basic parish nurse preparation course to our area. I accepted the offer to attend this course.

Parish nursing is a lot like starting a new business because you are creating something from nothing. During that first year, I listened actively to learn the needs, interests, and concerns of our parishioners. I also responded to requests for home, hospital, and nursing home visits, seeing over 150 individuals during the first two years.

We have since organized a group of health professionals within our church to perform quarterly blood pressure screenings. Several people have become more aware of unstable or elevated blood pressures and acted to correct this with their doctors. Last year, I recognized an urgent need to repeat a blood pressure screening on a woman who was completely unaware of her seriously elevated blood pressure until she participated at a church screening. It was 210/120 that morning, so I asked her permission to recheck her in her own home later that afternoon. I wanted to be in her normal environment for the repeat check. The second reading was still seriously elevated. I asked her to contact her doctor right then with the screening results. Her doctor started her on medication that night. It's been a little over a year since the follow-up screening. She told me recently that her blood pressure is being managed well with medications. Her other blood abnormalities have responded to medication. She exercises daily and has decided to retire from a very stressful job!

For the past two years we have raised breast cancer awareness by walking in the Susan G. Komen Race for the Cure. I started a breast cancer support group when a woman parishioner approached me after mass one weekend to tell me that she had just been diagnosed with breast cancer and needed help. She wanted support right here at church. I had never formed a support group before and felt a bit uncertain.

I immediately prayed to God for guidance and remembered that I had bought a resource book a year ago at the annual Parish Nurse Symposium. I started reading *Effective Support Groups—How to Plan, Design, Facilitate, and Enjoy Them,* by James E. Miller (1998). The simple guidelines reassured me. I have discovered that *". . . People come together seeking support. What they discover is that they have support to give as well as receive. They also discover a freedom to talk and an understanding acceptance that they may find hardly anywhere else, and perhaps at nowhere else."* [1]

The support group currently has six or seven women and a couple of husbands, out of a total of 16 members listed, who continue to meet monthly. The format for the support group is simple. We open with spontaneous prayer, light a candle, and then listen as the stories unfold. We close with a *Thanksgiving Litany,* a prayer that I found in *The Ligourian,* a catholic magazine published by the Redemptorist Order. I contacted their publisher and received copyright permission to make enough copies for us to use in the group. The *Thanksgiving Litany* has a positive focus and the group has embraced it.

Two members of our Breast Cancer Support Group are currently receiving chemotherapy. The woman who originally requested support a year ago has been diagnosed with liver metastasis. The other woman experienced a poor

---

[1] Miller, James E. *Effective Support Groups: How to Plan, Design, Facilitate, and Enjoy Them.* Fort Wayne: Willowgreen Publishing, 1998.

first diagnosis and treatment from her first doctor. Once she began to feel supported within the group, she decided to seek a second medical opinion. She consequently underwent a full single mastectomy for a reappearing aggressive cancer. Both of these women are struggling in so many ways—emotionally, spiritually and physically. They are gradually experiencing a connection to themselves and to others in the group that is comforting and healing. I am witnessing the development of courage and hope through the caring they are receiving and giving to each other. As the parish nurse I continue to facilitate the activity of the Breast Cancer Support Group. I feel inspired by them.

Chapter 87

Southern Belles

By Tracie Shields

I have taken care of many wonderful people over the course of my career. I can still recall many of their names and faces. One person in particular was Ms. Betty. She was a petite older lady—very quiet and very sweet. She was a "Southern Belle" to me (much like my mother), born and raised in the southern U.S. She was a great listener and would often ask the nurses about their families and boyfriends. Then she would listen and enjoy our stories. She never imparted much about her own life. I don't think she had any children. Her husband was a different story. He came in to see her for brief visits. He wasn't a very nice man and if it was nighttime, you could always smell the alcohol around him. I would ask her leading questions and try to listen to her, but she didn't choose to talk about herself.

Another patient who comes to mind when I think of Ms. Betty is Ms. Mary. Ms. Mary was also quite the "Southern Belle". She was like Ms. Betty in so many ways. She was also quiet and so kind to everyone who entered her room. She wasn't one to talk about herself, but was interested in everyone else's woes and was also a great listener. The difference was that Ms. Betty was Caucasian and Ms. Mary was African-American. One especially hectic night, I was in charge on the 3:00–11:00 pm shift. I received a call from the emergency room midway through the shift that Ms. Betty needed to be admitted. Her cancer was no longer responding to treatment and had spread into her lungs. There would be a hospice consult to follow the next day. I only had one bed available and it was in the room with Ms. Mary. The two had been patients at the same time, but had never been roommates. They hadn't even met each other. I knew they would get along great. My only concern was that Ms. Betty would most likely die and Ms. Mary was in the middle of her treatments. I tried to be sensitive to the patients as they battled their disease. I didn't want Ms. Mary demoralized by seeing the disease win.

I talked with Ms. Mary before Ms. Betty arrived. I explained that she would be getting a roommate whom she would really like, but that her new roommate was very ill. I probably would be moving her to a hospice bed the next day. Ms. Mary smiled and patted my hand. She said "Don't you worry about me. You just do what you need to do."

As we placed Ms. Betty in her bed, Ms. Mary looked on in sympathy. Ms. Betty's husband paced outside the door. I could smell the alcohol from inside the room. As I left the room, Ms. Mary and Ms. Betty were quietly exchanging words. I didn't hear exactly what was said, but it amazed me how they already seemed bonded. There was already an understanding between the two. I knew a friendship was blooming. I was not prepared, however, for what awaited me in the hallway.

Ms. Betty's husband was enraged. He nearly blew me over with his alcohol-saturated breath as he demanded that his wife be moved immediately. As I began to suspect why he demanded her moved, I also realized the danger of the situation. Although he was not an enormous man, I was in my early 20s and at 5'2" I weighed a little over 100 lbs. I knew what alcohol could do to an angry man. I slowly backed into the nurses' station, nearer to the phones. Once I was within hands-reach of the phone I realized it was time to "grow up" as a nurse and stand my ground. I had stood my ground many times with doctors, nurses, patients, and families, but this was the true test. I calmly informed the man that this was the only bed available for his wife. Due to the hospice consult, she would be moving to an available hospice room by morning. I asked him calmly to please leave the unit as visiting hours were over. He then screamed at me "I don't want my wife in that room with that woman overnight!"

Rather than fear, I was filled with rage and embarrassment for the ladies in their room. We were only a few feet away from Ms. Mary and Ms. Betty's room and everyone on the unit had heard his yelling. As call lights alarmed and nurses came running, I picked up the phone and paged security. I told him to leave before he was arrested for public intoxication. I walked into the room where Ms. Betty lay. She had her eyes closed and her breathing was shallow. Ms. Mary said "We're okay, child. I'll watch her because I can't sleep anyway. I'll hit the call light if anything changes. You go see about your other patients. We're okay."

I still meet people who I don't understand and I still run up against prejudice that I don't understand. But, I still remember two very dear ladies, very much mirror images of one another who shared their souls in a hospital room years ago. And I still remember their smiles.

CHAPTER 88

THE CALL I WILL NEVER FORGET

BY WENDELL ALDERSON

I've been a flight nurse for 11 years. I've learned to classify my calls in three ways. First are the calls you do not remember anything about. Even when you go back and read the chart, you still don't recall anything. Then come the calls you may not remember at first, but when you read your chart or talk with someone about the mission, your memory is jogged enough to recall the flight. Finally, there are calls you never forget. You remember every detail. These calls affect you emotionally and physically. You would like to forget them and place them into one of the first two categories, but, no matter what you do, they stay vivid in your memory. Hopefully, you learn to work through these calls and go on with your job and life, but the memories are always clear in your mind.

This call falls into the third category. Although this flight happened more than three years ago, I will never forget it. At 3:00 am, we were dispatched to a remote area in the foothills above Sacramento for a trailer fire. We had to land at a local sawmill and be transported to the scene in a police squad car over dirt roads. We were told that only one ambulance had reached the scene and that the fire had occurred in a campground. Upon hearing that information, we decided to take our pilot with us for an extra pair of hands.

We found three victims at the scene: a 2-year-old child with 60% burns, an adult man with 70% burns, and an adult woman with 70% burns. Only one advanced life support provider was on scene. The victims had been pulled from a fully involved trailer fire and were lying on the ground with their burned clothing on. The only lighting came from flashlights the other campers held for us.

The medic had intubated the man. The child and the women both required immediate airway management. We went to the child first. After establishing an intravenous line, we were able to give a short-acting paralytic and achieve an oral airway. We wrapped him in clean sheets and began ventilating him. After intubating the child, my partner was committed to staying with him.

The medic was already with the adult man managing his airway. Now was the time to get to the woman and provide the care she needed. The only person I had to help me was my pilot. I attempted a nasal airway without success. I found no intravenous access, and an oral airway was not possible because the patient's jaw was locked. My only option was to perform a surgical opening into the larynx. I had done them before, but always with my partner, another flight nurse.

I began the surgery with only the light from a flashlight being held by a camper I was sure was going to faint any minute. The procedure was difficult because of severe burns over the woman's neck area. My pilot was able to hold the patient's head still as I did the procedure. She also handed me the instruments I needed as I asked for them. She followed my directions well, and I credit her willingness to help.

By this time another ambulance had arrived on the scene. We loaded all three patients into the two ambulances and began the long drive back to the landing zone. When we arrived, two other helicopters were there along with ours. We gave report to the other flight teams and transferred care of the two adults to them. We kept the child with us.

All three patients were transported to the University of California-Davis Medical Center. The flight lasted about 20 minutes. The sun was just rising when we landed at the hospital. It had been a long night. After giving report on our patient to the trauma team, my partner and I went into the utility room and began to cry. Our emotions were overwhelming. In all my years as a flight nurse, this call is still my worst. We had several critical-incident stress de-briefings after the flight. I was off for several days, which was good.

CHAPTER 89

IN THE MIDDLE OF THE NIGHT

BY LAURIE L. WISE

It's two-thirty in the morning. I'm awake again, lying on my parents' all too un-comfortable couch, listening to what might be my father's last breaths. I am weary beyond weary, drained of tears and strength, missing my husband, feeling angry at my siblings, and bereft of any compassion or sympathy for my needy mother.

I am not the stellar picture of nursing excellence at this point, but I am, above all, still a nurse. I am caring for my father in his last weeks on earth. I am doing all the things I have been trained for, using skills and observations that are to me, like breathing. Why has nothing I've learned in 30 years of caring for others prepared me for this hardest of tasks?

To begin with, of course, I am not ready for him to die. This man, who has been the most important influence in my life, still has some influencing to do. I am still a streak of paint on an unfinished canvas. I need his touch, his wisdom, his vision. I need his presence and his laughter, his force, in my life. I am selfish beyond measure.

Knowing he's had a predictable, terminal illness has been both a blessing and a curse. For years now, we have known that as soon as he stopped his monthly, then bi-monthly, then weekly transfusions, that he would die. His bone marrow void of those all-important red cells would cease to function, and his life would end. The blessing comes from knowing, from sharing whatever thoughts and dreams are important to all of us, and spending treas-ured time with this man we all love. The curse has been honoring his choices that are not mine; succumbing to this overpowering grief and frustration in dealing with those petty end-of-life issues that I have counseled countless others with such glib intensity.

Now, I am the recipient of hospice's call. Now it is my family, my support system that is under scrutiny. Now, my brothers and sister become the players in this drama of death and dying. It is at once, horrible and final. I think perhaps it is payback for all those times I was not as sympathetic or kind as I could have been to those in my care.

I know too much and not enough about my father's illness. I take leave of work, and move into my parents' cramped mobile home. I become transport, housekeeping, and social services melded into one hapless countenance. Mostly, I am just a survivalist for the three long weeks before he dies.

While he is alive, I know all the things to do and yet I know nothing. I drag him to the bathroom to bathe in the shower chair. I feast my eyes on his wasted, precious skin and love every inch that I bathe. He tells me again and again "you are rubbing too hard. Please be gentle. My hair even hurts." I cry countless tears, grateful for the mist in this claustrophobic bathroom. I note his decreasing urine output. I ask this proud, private man about his bowel movements. I constantly bug him about pain. He cups my cheek with his feeble, cold hand and says, "the only pain I have is you, dear." My funny, brilliant father, going for the joke to the end.

I decide that he would benefit from gentle massage, for his wasted limbs are now aching and cramped. The therapist comes to the house, and my father cannot comprehend how she knew he would love this. He asks me again and again, "How does she know me? Did you arrange this?"

His macular degeneration long ago has robbed him of his vision, but he still attempts to watch everything. He asks my sister to come closer "so I can see your freckles." He talks football scores with my brother-in-law. He uses up daylight the way I use up tissue.

I pretend to be composed. I ask the 'right' questions of the hospice nurse. I know all the impending signs of death. I know to get my mother to the funeral home for arrangements to be made. I wait for my youngest brother's visit to do this, knowing that I am not strong enough. My mother nearly collapses from the strain, and I shake inside, nauseated and reeling in this comic book of a funeral home. I know to call the cousin he loves, and when she hears he is failing, she hangs up the phone, and drives two and a half hours to spend 15 minutes with him, making him laugh.

Why is this harder for me than the myriad of other deaths I have attended? I am using the same skills, the same words. I am relying on the same wisdom. Why am I not able to summon the tools that all my mentors have shared with me all these years? Every night, I hide in the bedroom. I call my husband and weep. I tell him over and over "I cannot do this, please come and get me." I am furious with him because he cannot hear the panic in my voice, because he won't rescue me, and because he cannot save my father. I hate talking to my friends. They have never seen me this weak. I'm the one they come to when they have to tell someone bad news. I'm the 'seasoned' oncology nurse who has life and death in perspective. I'm the one with the balance, the right words, the knowing grace.

Eventually, it all falls into place. I am afforded that peaceful heart we all read about. My husband arrives. On the final weekend, my brother is the one on the couch, listening to those last breaths, while I escape to a hotel with my rescuer. I fall onto the bed, holding onto him with three weeks worth of anguish at my fingertips.

The call comes at 7:30 the next morning. My brother's voice is panicked but controlled. He tells me, "You'd better come back right now." I race down the highway, and find my dad holding court with my mother and brother at his side. He tells me, "you'd better get all the kids together. I think today is the day." I know better. He is still coherent, making urine, and sustaining his blood pressure. I tell him that all the kids have been here. He looks at me with his morphine-clouded eyes and gives me the last loving look I will remember forever, and slips peacefully into unconsciousness, surrounded by love that knows no end.

Two days later, he leaves us. I am the only one in the room, perched at his feet, rubbing his wasted legs. My brother is fittingly asleep in my father's chair, already positioned to assume the vacuum my father will leave. My mother comes into the room minutes after he's taken his last breath, and the sorrowful ending to this man's splendid life begins.

Three years later, I am still trying to understand what this experience has meant to me and to others. I know that the way I care for each of my patients changed the moment he died. It's as if the reservoir emptied by his life is somehow filled up by caring for all the people God has since sent my way. I know that I am a better nurse, a better sister, an improved but highly imperfect daughter, and a mighty warrior in honoring his precious life.

CHAPTER 90

MOTHERING MOTHER

BY NIKKI ODANGO ONGTAWCO

Three years ago on Mother's Day, I spent the day at my mother's hospital bedside. It was the first time she was away from home on that special occasion. But from the time she was admitted to the hospital in May 2000, she was never alone—her twelve children took turns at her side.

She survived surgery to repair an aortic aneurysm and lung failure. She was subsequently supported by mechanical ventilation. Weaning her from the ventilator machine was unsuccessful. My mother wanted to come home to attend special affairs, cook her favorite food for us, or spend holidays with her grandchildren. As a daughter and a nurse, I was devastated, for I knew her chances of coming home were slim to none. I focused on her welfare from that moment. With the help of my husband, whose specialty is cardiac care, my family was able to recognize the seriousness of her condition.

After several months in the hospital, the doctors recommended a transfer to a highly skilled nursing facility, as she was still on the ventilator. My family and I faced a dilemma: Would our mother hate us if we placed her in a nursing home? In our Asian culture we take care of our ailing parents when they can no longer take care of themselves. From what I observed in the area where we live, very seldom would one encounter an Asian person in a nursing home. It was not quite acceptable that our parents be placed in that kind of setting. We pondered the pros and cons of our decision. Ultimately, it was our mother who encouraged us to do the best thing for her.

When she settled in her new 'home,' I had to plan my schedule strategically since I worked full-time during the week in an obstetrics/gynecology office and part-time at a local hospital on weekends. Every minute of my life was crucial in those three years considering I also had to look after my mother-in-law, who had a heart-bypass surgery.

When my mom began her rehabilitation, I told her that a long journey begins with one step. She had to learn the basics all over again: taking steps, grasping objects, eating, swallowing, talking, and eventually breathing on her own. I studied her condition and researched every possible way to make this transition easier for everyone. Caring for her was different from what I was used to in my regular nursing role. With the help of my family, we were able to achieve our goal—to get her to try living again. After grueling weeks of determination and persistence, she was able to master those tasks with ease, to the point that she was able to go back to doing her favorite activities, such as cross-stitching, writing, reading, and watching her favorite soaps.

As the days progressed, my mother's care required more attention. I made sure that she understood the plan of care discussed during doctors' rounds and encouraged her to write down any concerns or problems she had. The whole family made changes in their schedules to accommodate her needs. It was not easy in the beginning, especially when everyone had to work and care for their own families. We eventually scheduled a daily 'shift' for each one of us. We brought her favorite home-cooked food, changed her bed, combed her hair, prepared her clothes for the next day, transferred her to bed for the night, and ensured that her necessities were within reach. Eventually, all of us, including my brothers, learned to perform some of the duties that were once regarded as 'nursing chores,' like massaging her bony prominences and checking for any skin breakdown, changing her clothing, assisting when nature called, and most importantly, assessing her mental status.

Even her grandchildren became a familiar sight at the nursing center. They spent time with their "Nanay" any way they knew how: resting on her bed, doing their homework, eating junk foods she refused to eat, watching *Golden Girls* with her or a *Lifetime* original movie, or by simply sitting in a chair close to her. She gave them advice on school, love, or anything they wished to talk about. The children were not scared of seeing residents or patients on ventilators. They even befriended some of the residents and sat with them figuring out puzzles or just chatting about anything. These children were aware that those patients could have a good life while residing there if given proper care and love. So in essence, my mom enjoyed the quality of her life during the time spent in the nursing facility.

This was a woman whom the doctors said may not live long after major surgeries on her aorta and lungs. As with any surgery, they could not guarantee her quality of life afterward. But how do you define quality of life? I firmly believe that because of our vigilant approach to her care, she was able to live the last three years of her life comfortably and prepare herself for the next journey. Until the end, she enjoyed the only thing that mattered to her: to be surrounded by her family.

In the last few months before her death, my role as a nurse became more important, but my duty as her daughter became much stronger. I was torn between letting go and believing her life was still worth fighting for. The medical reports and tests indicated to me that I had to prepare the entire family for the inevitable. Some of my siblings felt there was still hope and others felt she was ready to go.

At the end of my mother's journey, I knew with all my heart that she received excellent care from each one of her children, far and near, and was showered with love and affection by her twenty-six grandchildren. The night before her passing, I watched her say goodbye to our oldest brother. Her departure was very difficult for the entire family, but we knew she was ready. Our mother had a very special way that warmed our hearts and left each one of us with beautiful memories.

CHAPTER 91

THE GIFT

BY TONI L. PHILLIPS

Sometimes we receive gifts and don't recognize the value of the gift until it presents itself within a new experience and we see it in a different light. This was the situation with me approximately six months after I received my RN license. At this early point in my new career, I felt a steady surge of confidence. I had strong clinical and organizational skills, and I was ready to apply my knowledge base. I really believed I knew what I was doing, and truly believed I was a *real nurse*.

One day, I was sharing my profound feelings of being a real nurse with a nursing assistant that I was working with on the 7:00 am to 3:00 pm shifts. The nursing assistant said to me, "You will truly be a nurse when you shed your first tear." Well, at the time I was insulted by the comment, and just figured that the nursing assistant didn't possess the qualifications or the educational back-ground to identify the characteristics of a true nurse. Therefore, I ignored her comment and continued to enjoy my increased autonomy and confidence within the nursing profession. Unfortunately, I wasn't bright enough to realize I was being given a gift.

One evening, on the 3:00 pm to 11:00 pm shift, I was assigned a 53-year-old woman with metastatic pancreatic cancer. There were lesions in the brain, spine, ribs, liver, kidney, and abdomen. I knew this diagnosis was grave, but up to this point in my six-month career, I hadn't personally cared for a dying patient. If this were to happen today, there would be several disciplines involved in her plan of care, but 20 years ago, it was only the social worker, the doctor, the family, and me. We didn't hastily discharge her from the hospital, but then we also didn't realize how quickly this disease would consume her life. Each day I came to work, I watched a wonderful young woman be consumed by a tragic disease process. Each day I wanted to care for this client to let her suffer a little less. Each day I wanted to help a family say good-bye to a family member that they were not ready to let go. Even though this client's physical appearance and internal structures deteriorated rapidly, her desire to care for others never ceased, despite her pain. This client embraced her death with a grace and style that illuminated the spirit of those around her.

I had the privilege to be at the bedside holding her hand when she died, on the 3-11 shift. I began to cry as the tears fell into both our hands and washed away the pain. It was at this moment I remembered what the nursing assistant had told me a few months earlier. "When you shed your first tear, you will truly be a nurse." Then I understood the special gift the nursing assistant had given me that I chose to ignore prior to caring for this patient. She was telling me about a critical part of nursing that can only be experienced, it can't be taught. You will know when it happens, because it touches your heart. Fortunately for me, this lesson manifested itself early in my career. Then I could reap the rewards of having my heart touched on a daily basis. I now share this valuable gift with my students, so their hearts will be warmed by their caring practices. I will always be grateful to that nursing assistant for her wisdom and for giving me this special gift, especially since the nursing assistant happened to be my mom. Thanks for the gift mom!

CHAPTER 92

ON ANGELS' WINGS

BY DONNA M. NICKITAS

It was early New Year's morning when the phone rang and woke me from a sound sleep. The voice on the other end was the nurse, Mary, from the nursing home informing me that my mother's condition had worsened. Her breathing was slowing, skin was mottling, and death was impending. Mom's condition began to fail right after Christmas. Her body could no longer stage off the respiratory infection or her mind find the willpower to fight it back. I realized the temperature from inside her caused the heat to burn right through her body into my hand. It was as though the heat ignited a flame—a flame that revealed to me the level of pain and suffering she was enduring.

As I touched my mother's brow and looked deeply into her blue eyes, I knew the time had come for me to release her from this body, a body overcome by infection. It was my mother's time to go—the right time, the perfect time. This realization about timing would set into motion the most difficult decision I ever needed to make. As my mother's power of attorney and health care proxy, I would inform her physician that I knew my mother's condition would not improve and it was time to intervene. Together, we reviewed her care plan and decided to stop the tube feedings and start the morphine. With her health care needs addressed, I sought my sister's help to address Mom's spiritual needs. She would call the social worker and arrange for the priest to give my mother a final blessing. As I stood at the foot of the bed, I realized I was in a role I knew so well—giving orders, setting priorities, and organizing activities. The nurse inside me knew just what to do. The daughter in me needed to take hold and understand what message I was sending to my mother, my sister, and, most importantly, to myself. This message was one of peace. I was willing to release my mother in peace and total trust to the expert care of angels. I had come to accept the timing of the universe and that it was perfectly fine to prepare for death.

My mother allowed her family enough time to prepare for her impending death. She was stubborn like that. It was always her way or the highway. So when the phone call came telling me about my mother's impending death, I understood that the message that was delivered firmly but compassionately as only a nurse could. The nurse in me knew that I had to proceed quickly, for my Mom would not make it through the day. As I gathered my strength to inform my children about their grandmother, I knew I had to go quickly to be at my mother's bedside. My greatest fear was that she would die alone with no one there to comfort and support her. I forced myself to stay calm and hasten the children to dress. I kept speaking to my mother aloud and telling her I was on the way. Out the door and in the car, I started to prepare myself for the role that I have prepared so many of my nursing students to take on.

As a nurse educator, I have taught several lessons on how to comfort and console the dying and support the family during the process. First and foremost, I remember the fear and anxiety in the faces of my nursing students as I discussed the concept of death. For many of them, death was a foreign concept, one that they had no personal experience with. Thus it was one of the most challenging tasks of my teaching career. I often required students to reflect upon the meaning of death and describe how they would like to die.

As I read these reflections, I began to fully understand why students were afraid to learn about death and more importantly why they needed to express their fears openly. Death was viewed as the end of life, a final event. To me, grasping the meaning of death was to accept the fact that death was actually a part of life. Although all knew this truth about death, each student indeed had not accepted it. Up to this point, death had not been addressed in the nursing curriculum; no one even dared to mention the "D" word. Were nursing students really responsible for knowing about death and dying or end of life care? Of course most nurses would respond by saying 'yes.' I first introduce the topic of death, dying, and spirituality into a course entitled Introduction to Nursing. My intent is to have nursing students understand that death is not something to be feared, and, more importantly, to prepare future nurses to care for the dying.

Now I was no longer teaching about caring for the dying but rather preparing myself to care for my own mother. By the time my family and I arrived at the nursing home, I had reflected upon those lessons I taught on death and dying. Suddenly, those lessons came back with vividness and insight like no others before. I quickly realized that I had to leave the nurse at the door of my mother's room and enter as the daughter I was. As much as the nurse in me wanted to reposition her body, clear her airway, and cool my mother's brow with a soft wash cloth, the daughter in me just held her hand and whispered words of love and support. It was in these last moments together that we confirmed our eternal love—a love between a mother and child. A lifetime of memories filled the space between our hands and a prayer on our lips allowed us to experience a moment of peace and grace.

In the presence of my children, husband, and other family members we watched as each breath my mother took became more labored than the one before. Death let its presence be known as her skin became cooler and cooler to the touch. There was no more pain and suffering to be had, and in the last seconds angels arrived as the birds chirped loudly in the courtyard to carry my mother to her eternal resting place. This place, I believe, is filled with love, where pain and suffering no longer exist. Although my mother left on New Year's Day on angels' wings, I know the daughter she left behind will celebrate life with full recognition that a mother's work is never done—it just transforms and becomes the work that daughters do.

CHAPTER 93

ALICE: THE LESSONS GO ON

BY MARY ALICE CASH

A young nursing student, two weeks away from graduation, came up to me the other day. "I never thought I could work in a nursing home, she said, "until I met your mom." She goes on. "She calls me by name, thanks me for every thing I do for her, she even remembers my children's names and it's been a year since I told her!"

I choke back the tears as a swell of love and pride overcomes me. "I wish you had known her when she was a nurse," I respond. "Mom has made more of an impact on people since the day she stopped nursing than she did when she was working."

My mom, Alice, always dreamed of being a nurse. Responsibility and caring for others came naturally to her. As one of the oldest children in a family of twelve, she grew up in a rural home during the depression. She studied hard and managed to graduate as salutatorian of her class, securing her a place in nursing school.

But, as with many families at the time, finances were such that she could not attend. Disappointed but undaunted, she began working in a factory. Eventually, she met my dad, fell in love, and married. With marriage came the added responsibilities of caring for a live-in, diabetic, senile mother-in-law and an alcoholic father-in-law. Three children came along and it seemed she would never fulfill her dream.

When the children were all in school, and her mother-in-law had passed away, she heard of a practical nursing program, applied, and was accepted. It looked like Mom was on her way! Soothing the ego of a husband who was insecure about his wife joining the work force, she secured a position at the area psychiatric hospital. At forty years of age, when many people were at the high point of their careers, Mom was just starting hers. She wanted more! The dream of being a registered nurse had been rekindled.

She found a way to manage nursing school, despite a full time job and family. She worked the night shift at the hospital, drove forty miles every day to college, and studied every spare moment. I don't remember ever missing a meal, or not seeing her sparkling eyes brimming with pride at all of our school events. After two long years she graduated as a registered nurse, never missing a beat as wife, mother, or friend. My dad cried as she walked across the stage to finally accept something that signified all the struggles and stumbling blocks that she had encountered and overcome. At that moment we were overwhelmed with love's pride as each of us shared in her achievement. My mom, the nurse!

She was a wonderful nurse. People with that much determination are seldom mediocre. She continued to work at the psychiatric hospital and her building housed many elderly men and women patients, long forgotten and forsaken by their families. My friends and I would stop by occasionally to visit. You always knew which ward Mom worked on. The patients were nicely dressed. Ladies' hair was combed and curled. Men were neatly shaven, beds were fresh, and floors were mopped—all the extra things not taught in textbooks. She would proudly introduce each patient to us as though they were honored ambassadors. Their eyes would glimmer when she spoke to them. They'd smile their toothless smiles, with tongues rolling from the side effects of their medications, and reach out to her. She would always hug them, talk to them, and gently caress their heads and hands. She saw them for what they really were—human beings in need of love and attention.

It was during these years that she took one brief leave of absence. Dad had cancer. She cared for him at home, keeping him comfortable at a time before chemotherapy and hospice were available. After a two-month battle, he died peacefully and with dignity. She returned to work and eventually was promoted to supervisor. By now, the grandchildren had started arriving in her life and she began to look forward to retirement and travel.

One afternoon while getting ready for work, Mom decided to hang a plant on the back porch. Climbing a step stool, she lost her balance and fell over the porch rail. It was not much of a fall, but the results were devastating nonetheless. The impact resulted in a severed spinal cord and permanent paralysis—a truly life-changing experience for everyone whose lives she had touched. As another stumbling block faced her, she met the challenge, adjusted her life, and taught us how to assist her and accept change. She made us all stronger as a result of her tenacity and determination.

In the years since mom's accident, I have been approached by many people, professional and non-professional, who say things like "I was hanging curtains the other day and thought of your mom. I got down off the chair and waited for help." Or, " I was climbing a ladder the other day, leaned over too far, thought of your mom, got down and readjusted the ladder." Those who remember my mom have brought many precarious events to my attention. Because of her unfortunate accident, they stop what they are doing and make safer choices.

Mom lives in a nursing home now. It's not the retirement she had dreamed of; the only travel now is to the dining room by wheelchair. Yet every day she shows nurses and others that, while a diploma and a uniform may be the outward signs of being a nurse, even without these, you can go on appreciating each other's humanity from your own quiet little place.

CHAPTER 94

PARTY TALK

BY PATRICE RANCOUR

I'm mingling at a party. When people hear that I work at a cancer hospital, the most common inquiry is "Isn't that depressing? Working with all those dying people—how can you stand it?"

Most commonly, I respond with a question such as, "when you leave work at the end of the day, do you notice the way the light filters through the trees?" Or, "do you bury your nose in your kid's hair when you go home, just to smell it?" Or better yet, I tell a story that begins with another question. "When was the last time someone at work prayed for you?"

* * *

The room is spun with love as I quietly enter. There is a death watch being held here. Numerous friends and family members surround the bed of a forty-year-old man; husband, father of three babies. The cocoon they have woven around him is palpable and filled with their warmth and tenderness. Everyone should die in such an embrace as this.

They watch silently as I approach the bed, touch his arm and whisper my name into his comatose ear. I tell him he is surrounded by all those who cherish him and that all have given him their blessing to do whatever he needs to do next, whatever the next right step is for him.

As I step away from the bed, I inquire as to how it goes with the vigil-keepers. After some talk, I perceive it is time for me to withdraw and give this group the privacy they require. Before I leave, the dying man's sister asks me, "Is this what you do all day here?" I reply that it is part of my work. "Would it be alright," she says, " if we said a prayer for you?" And as a tear slides down my cheek, the group holds hands, bow their heads, and I too am woven into the tapestry of their embrace.

* * *

"Tell me," I say at the party to the person who is now looking at me oddly, "When was the last time at work you were privy to an experience of absolute ecstasy?"

* * *

The fifty-four-year-old man had been failing for some time. His wife, daughter, and son-in-law had finally stopped their cheerleading and were now available to him in another capacity. One Sunday morning, early, he awoke and begged his wife to "please turn off that light—it is so blinding, I can hardly bear it."

"But Richard, there is no light on, honey. It's 3:30 in the morning."

But the man lay with his arms across his face reporting that the light in the room was so dazzling, he felt blinded. Later the same morning he woke again and was uncharacteristically energetic. "It's time to call everyone in today. I don't have much time. I want to say good-bye."

And so his wife did. That Sunday afternoon, as he held court, his visitors remarked on the light that shone from him. Toward evening, he lost his energy, the light dimmed, and, as the room cleared, he began to lapse into sleep. As he did so, he beckoned to his son-in-law and fought to whisper his last words: "Now don't forget, you'll find it between the third and fourth trees."

His son-in-law was puzzled. "Dick, what are you talking about? What trees?" But the man merely repeated his statement before he quietly slipped away, never to reawaken. The next day his wife and son-in-law kept an appointment they had made at the cemetery to pick out a double plot. She was expressing her disappointment to the cemetery representative. Her husband had wanted to be buried under trees and it was unfortunate that there was no such double plot available.

"Well, it's funny you should mention that, ma'am," he returned. "Just this morning, a couple withdrew their reservation for a double plot in another section. I can take you there now, if you'd like." And as he pulled around the knoll and came to a slow stop in front of the site, the son-in-law clasped her arm.

"My God, Margaret," he whispered. "Dick saw this."

"Well that's ridiculous," she replied. "How could he have? We're just seeing it for the first time now." Nonetheless, they stared at the double plot site nestled in a grove of old oaks that filed past them. It was a plot between the third and fourth trees.

* * *

The party-goer takes a sip and looks at me warily, but I am relentless now. "When was the last time someone at work—a total stranger—let you into the most intimate moment of her life?"

* * *

The older woman is distraught as she sits in front of me. The problem is not the incurable pancreatic cancer she was diagnosed with six months ago. At that time, she was encouraged to "get your affairs in order." She did so in addition to taking a standard course of chemotherapy that was not expected to do much for her, but was offered as an option nonetheless.

At the time of her diagnosis, she had been married for thirty years to a man who had been neglectful of her. She had been miserable in this marriage and confessed to me that she had understood her diagnosis as a blessing, a legitimate way out of a difficult situation.

Surprisingly, however, her husband was awakened by the news of her diagnosis and was devastated by it. He became obsessively devoted to her and could not do enough for her. She basked in his tenderness, which she had never before experienced, even as a bride. When, six months later, a scan proclaimed her as having no evidence of disease, her physician scratched his head, chalked it up to 'spontaneous remission' and gave her a clean bill of health.

Her husband once again reverted to his old behavior and she now sits in disbelief in front of me. She has been once again sentenced to a life of abject lovelessness.

I turn to her and ask, "Must you once more resort to dying for your husband's attention?" I turn to her husband who sits in front of me, detached, and ask, "Can you not see how powerfully healing your love is?"

* * *

I regale the party-goer with one more anecdote despite his obvious chaffing.

* * *

The room is dark. I can barely see into it. I do detect movement, though. There is a woman on the bed writhing, her spirit is anguished. A man, her husband, is pacing frantically as he watches his wife's agony and feels powerless before it.

This is the first time I meet this couple. He informs me that she has just had the linings of her lungs sclerosed; that is, scarred together by a chemical agent. This prevents them from filling with fluid repeatedly, a not unusual complication for some cancer patients. Unfortunately, her analgesic premedications have not kicked in yet and she is in great pain.

The Buddhists have a wonderful saying: "It is easy to keep your heart open in heaven. It is so much harder to keep your heart open in hell." This woman must feel like she's in hell.

I move to the head of the bed and ask, "On a scale of 0 to 10, 0 being no pain, 10 being the worst pain imaginable, how would you rate your pain right now?"

She says through clenched teeth, "Honey, it doesn't even show up on your scale." Her husband looks at me in panic.

I quietly lower myself to her ear and say softly, "Come, breathe with me." And as we begin to breathe together, I take her on a voyage through her body, inviting her to inhale a soothing light with each breath that coolly puffs its way into each part of her body. Within ten minutes we have reduced pain intensity to a "5." And within twenty minutes, she is sleeping. The husband escorts me out of the room where we meet a group of white lab coats entering. "No," he says to them quietly. "It is enough." He turns them away at the door.

* * *

The party-goer chews the hors d'oevre nervously, silently, apparently regretful about having asked me about my work. Regardless, I say, "You see, my work is not about dying. It's about living." And as he turns away, I add, "Oh, and don't forget to bury your nose in your kid's hair when you get home tonight and find her sleeping. Just let yourself inhale the fragrance of it. I guarantee, you won't be sorry."

CHAPTER 95

MUTUAL SUPPORT

BY ALICE FACENTE

I always had a million excuses why I didn't go back to school for a master's degree in nursing. But I couldn't think of one good excuse when Margie asked me why I hadn't pursued that dream. Margie stopped me dead in my tracks. She was completely bald except for a few strands of hair that hadn't fallen out from her chemotherapy treatments. She had a swollen belly, ghostly pale skin, grossly swollen ankles and feet, and could hardly stand. She had a bucket nearby to catch unexpected bouts of vomiting. Still, she had a smile on her face. The question she had asked me was simple enough: "What are your plans for your future in nursing?" What possible excuse could I invent to tell this courageous lady why I hadn't gone back to school? Every excuse seemed feeble when I thought about the ordeal Margie had gone through, and what we both knew lay ahead.

She had cancer of the heart, a rarity even at the large teaching hospital in CT where the diagnosis was first made; only the second person with that diagnosis in 20 years. There could be no surgery, but a chemotherapy protocol was designed to shrink the growing tumor in the atrium of her heart. Chemotherapy would bring her almost to the brink of death, then let her 'rest' for two weeks before starting the next round. She was at one of the lowest points of her treatment when I first became her visiting nurse. I admitted her to home care services for daily injections of a medicine that would boost her white blood cells. These were the same type of vital, infection-fighting white blood cells that were being inadvertently destroyed by the chemo.

That day, I couldn't answer Margie when she asked me why I had not gone back to school like I said I always wanted to. That same day, I went home and called the local university and inquired about their graduate program in nursing. I would be too embarrassed to return to Margie's house the next day and say that I had no time to start pursuing my goal!

I wrote up my application for graduate school and mailed it within the week. I started school three months later, nervous as a kitten in a dog pound. I had graduated from nursing school 25 years earlier, and was sure that I was much too old to juggle work, raise a family, and attend graduate school. But every time I felt overwhelmed, I would get a mental image of Margie's bald head and think of her much more difficult battle. For the next few months, I would go to Margie's house in the morning, give her the painful injection, and then briefly update her on my school activities, projects, and papers. She enjoyed hearing my juggling antics, but also reveled in my successes, like when I received an "A" in my first course.

Margie's husband, Paul, was several years older than her 69 years, and although he wanted to help her, he was relieved to defer the nursing care to us visiting nurses. As it was, he was the one who now had to assume household responsibilities that Margie was too weak to do. Paul soon learned to make a mean vegetable soup from scratch!

My husband and children were very supportive of my educational pursuit, and the changes my schoolwork brought to our family life, but I learned in my second course that Margie was my true ally. We all need an ally to propel us forward into a life-changing event. She was the one who enabled me to forget all excuses and enthusiastically cheered me on when I faltered.

Soon Margie's health started to improve, and after her last round of chemotherapy, she no longer needed my assistance. Margie was very grateful for the help she received from the nurses when she was so gravely ill and weak. I was happy to be able to discharge her from home care services due to improved health. For the next year or so, I continued to work hard at my studies as well as work full-time as a nurse. Margie continued to improve, and I would see her occasionally in town, with a full head of short, wavy, white hair and skinny ankles and feet!

But about a year later, the cancer returned with a vengeance. This time she was unprepared to fight it as ferociously as before. She had a stem-cell transplant, a drastic procedure, and one that she and her family felt was a last-ditch effort to stop the spread of the cancer. Meanwhile, I was working hard in my nursing courses, and could see my graduation in sight.

Then came the call that Margie needed home care again, but this time the message from the hospital discharge planner was that she was dying, and was to be kept comfortable at home. Her devoted family was heartbroken. Paul was a good husband, by now used to doing all of the needed household chores, but he looked to his daughter-in-law and me to help him attend to Margie's personal care needs.

Like so many older men, Paul was embarrassed to do any personal care for his wife, but he was willing to learn to do anything necessary to make her comfortable. I taught Paul to change her bed linens with Margie still in it, rolling her side-to-side. I brought a commode for him to lift her onto whenever she needed to use it. I taught him about incontinence briefs, which he learned how to change quickly and discreetly. I taught him about liquid pain medication that he needed to administer for her comfort. Together we bathed her in bed, changed her clothes, and made her comfortable in her last days.

Margie died peacefully in her own bed, with her beloved husband at her side. She was my ally for pursuing my dream of graduate school, and I felt I was her ally in enabling her to have a dignified end-of-life experience at home. Helping her husband accomplish that was my payback for her enthusiasm and support.

One year later, I graduated with honors with a master's degree in nursing. My husband, children, and mother stood proudly in the crowd when I received my degree. I truly felt that one other person, my ally Margie, was looking down proudly from heaven that day, too, cheering me on as always.

CHAPTER 96

THOUGHTS AT THE END OF THE DAY

BY SHELLEY B. ADAMS

There are many reasons for feeling good at the end of your day. Whether the dog bounds eagerly toward you upon walking in your house, or you caught the last glimpse of the sunset and remember that you left home as it arose. Maybe it's slipping into the warmth of your bed after the unexpected double shift or feeling the arms of your loved ones embrace you before you can take off your coat. Everyone has his or her own interpretation of what feels good at the end of the day.

I graduated from nursing school over 20 years ago. This is not such an awe-inspiring statement, except that I am different from most of the nurses I have known who had dreams of being a nurse from a very early age. Not only did I never consider being a nurse, but I was almost convinced by my aunt (who was a nurse) to not take that path.

So, why did I choose nursing? I still cannot answer that question, other than to say that it makes me feel good at the end of my day. For some unknown reason, I chose to change my major one afternoon in the dormitory. I was living with a few nursing students and could not get enough of their discussions about what they were doing in class and clinical sites.

By now I've done a little of everything. I know enough to handle difficult situations in any setting and am contemplating a higher degree. I am a nursing director in behavioral health, one of the many areas I originally thought to be not my cup of tea and shied away from. Of course, the same was true for long-term care, office settings, emergency rooms, surgery, nurseries, medical-surgical floors, and so on. It's not just a morbid curiosity that sent me in each direction. For lack of a better way to explain, it's my own fear of missing out on something! This may not come as a comfort to the hundreds of patients I've cared for, the many supervisors who have rated me, or the instructors who have taught me, but give me a moment to explain myself.

I have always been in motion. I find that if I sit too long, sleep too long, or stay in one place too long there is a growing urgency to seek what I am missing. Having given up a potential journalism career (I began college on a journalism scholarship) and early thoughts of becoming a policewoman, I am thankful that nursing came to me. There is really no excuse to be bored in the workplace! Nurses can do a variety of tasks in innumerable settings.

Whenever I found that I was weary from technology I changed to a setting that offered a more human touch. If I found my body to be worn at the end of the day, I found a position that called more upon my intellect. There have been times when I exhausted all parts of my being, and times I felt not challenged enough.

The one common link to my varied experiences is how I felt at the end of each day. It is as if God let me in on one of his many secrets. I always found that I touched someone every day of my life, be it patient, client, resident, colleague, student, friend, or family member. I have been heard saying to interviewees and students that we, as nurses, have the uncanny ability to sell ourselves every day. We greet the people we care for, ill and well, and without effort, convince them to allow our hands to touch them, our voices to soothe them, and our hearts to love them.

I have walked miles of long hallways and sat in many a tiresome meeting. I have guided a baby from the womb and laid it in its mother's arms. I have held the hand of a dying man as he drew his last breath. I have medicated the terminal patient and held his wife as she cried. I have turned and bathed comatose patients who never looked into my eyes. There have been the tearful children who agreed after the injection, "that wasn't so bad!" I have listened to countless life stories of the aged and been called an angel just for walking into their rooms.

Ask me how I felt at the end of these days. I am ceaselessly amazed that no matter how dreary the outcomes or how miraculous the recoveries, I was a part of someone's life and played a role I never could have if not a nurse. The greatest gifts a nurse receives are felt forever. The smile from the patient who is told, "The doctor said you could be discharged today!" The hand you held that squeezed yours tightly out of fear. "Thank God you are here," when offering pain medication. And maybe just, "I'm so glad you made time to talk to me."

I believe we are chosen to follow the road God paves before us. For every tear I have shed when I have lost a patient, it eventually came to soothe me. For every day I felt like I would never make it through one more chart, a suffering person's moan reminded me that I had the strength to go on. In every selfish, human moment of thinking, 'why am I doing this?' someone is sent to tell me how much the little girl in the room at the end of the hall enjoyed the silly story I told her.

How do you feel at the end of your day? Can you keep track of the smiles you have found as you wiped away tears? Do you remember the struggles for life that ended in peaceful slumber? How many times have you been told, "I never could have made it without you"?

I can tell you how I feel at the end of my day. There is a sense of worth for having contributed to someone's life. There is a memory created from a new encounter. There is a rich blessing in knowing that, no matter how minor the deed, I assisted or educated a person who was in need. What other profession could offer me the opportunity to touch people in so many ways? Being a nurse makes me feel good at the end of my day, as I am certain it will at the end of my life.

CHAPTER 97

A FINE ART

By E. Rosellen Dedlow

When I was five, I learned to read. One of the first books I read was *Run Away, Little Girl* by Marilyn Segal. Afterward I told my mother I would grow up and take care of children like the little girl with cerebral palsy. There was no way for my mother to know then that I would be a nurse for children with special health care needs. There is also no earthly explanation for the series of events and people that helped shape that decision and my nursing practice today.

For example, in sixth grade, a friend and I read *The Miracle Worker* by William Gibson, the life story of Helen Keller. We decided to learn sign language because we kept getting in trouble for talking during class. We signed to each other surreptitiously over the course of the school year. Later that year, my family moved, and down the street lived a girl who was deaf. She and I could communicate because of my previous practice in sign language. I learned to value her as a friend, and see how she was like me instead of seeing her differences.

In high school in the 70s, I had a friend with spina bifida. Randy was in a wheelchair but was active and fun to be with. He lifted weights and went deep sea fishing. We enjoyed movies, road trips, and target practice at the local range. I remember a time when there were race riots at the high school, and fighting broke out in the halls. Randy came through the melee, swinging his wheelchair armrest widely, clearing a path through the crowd. He was determined to get me out of the school safely. I learned so many things from Randy: colostomies and pressure sores, the hurtfulness of teasing, how to load a wheelchair in a small car, the problems with inaccessible buildings, having a positive attitude in the face of adversity, and the importance of support from a devoted family.

As a Girl Scout, I camped and worked on community service projects. I earned the usual camping and cooking badges, but also earned child care and first aid badges. I loved working with younger girls in troops and camps. As a Senior Girl Scout, I pursued my First Class Award (the highest award a Girl Scout can earn). The requirements included community service projects in several areas and exploration of possible careers. Since I was interested in working with children, I spent one school year as a teacher's aide in a special education classroom deciding if I wanted to be a teacher. I spent a year as a volunteer ambulance driver considering whether I wanted to enter the health field from the high-adrenaline side of emergency care. Finally, I spent a year as a candy-striper in a local hospital. I loved the hospital setting, and my experience sealed the deal: I would be a nurse.

I went off to school at the local community college, got married, and graduated from nursing school. I worked in a small community hospital. I worked med-surg, geriatrics, ortho, cardiac, and other floors just waiting for a pediatric position to open up. When it did, I was overjoyed. I loved nights on the pediatric floor, rocking babies, holding little ones' hands, hearing bedtime prayers, settling moms and dads in to sleep beside their children. Even now, 20 years later, I remember certain children and moments that were special.

In spite of our wish to have children of our own, my husband and I have been unable to have children, so we enrolled as foster care parents. We had a series of wonderful experiences, culminating in the arrival of Nathan. Nathan needed a home that could provide special care because he had a breathing tube, and a feeding tube into his stomach. Nathan stayed with us for three wonderful years. I learned so much about caring for children with special needs, providing stimulation to help development, rejoicing in the small victories, and advocating for the best for my child.

We were thrilled to see Nathan progress, but I was devastated when circumstances dictated that Nathan be adopted out of state. This loss and other issues triggered a long battle with depression. I felt that I was put on this earth to work with children, but my sad and depressed mind figured that I had done my part with Nathan and life was over—no more children needed me. Years of struggling against the darkness of depression followed.

Then Patty arrived. My niece was born with low muscle tone, and had to be placed on a ventilator because she was too weak to breathe. She was hospitalized in a children's hospital five hours away from home. Her parents needed to keep working to maintain her health insurance and could not be where they wanted to be—at her bedside. Since I was then disabled by the depression, and not working, I went to stay with Patty for them. In the months that followed, I learned what it was like to talk to the teams of doctors, to spend night after night sleeping on the pediatric intensive care unit waiting room floor, and to watch a child struggle to survive. I met and shared with many other families spending long hours in the waiting room. I watched the PICU nurses and doctors as they cared for very sick children.

Patty helped me remember my calling. I noticed the difference in caring for an acutely ill child with a curable condition, and caring for a developmentally disabled or chronically ill child. I saw a focus on the illness, and a desperate need for focusing on health. I wanted to advocate for overcoming disability by reducing impairment, encouraging activities, and participation in life. When Patty went home on a ventilator with home care nursing, I experienced the trials that families go through with home care nursing and long-term care. I decided to return to school to become a nurse practitioner who would specialize in the care of children with special health care needs. I attended the University of Florida, receiving a dual degree as a clinical nurse specialist and pediatric nurse practitioner.

Patty died from an infection contracted during an unplanned admission. An error in the state Medicaid billing system delayed payment to the home care nursing company, and they could no longer provide home care. Although Patty was stable when she entered the hospital, she contracted a deadly respiratory virus and died of complications. After such an unnecessary loss, I knew I had to become a child health advocate for social and political issues, as well as health issues.

Life continued to place motivational people in my path. A college roommate, Carol, had cerebral palsy but was majoring in physical education. She was (and continues to be) one of the most upbeat, determined, and inspirational people I know. I found myself in the perfect place for finding my dream job and a system full of children who needed me. A local pediatrician was developing a program to coordinate the home care of technologically-dependent children. I became the pediatric nurse practitioner for the spina bifida clinic, the craniofacial clinic, the child development clinic, and the pediatric care coordination program. I began doing primary care for complex children, case management for special needs populations, assessments and feeding instruction for new parents of infants with cleft palates, and home care instruction for medically-complex children. I began educating patients, families, community providers, and health professionals. I began advocating for children politically and professionally. Although I found myself developing expertise in many areas, I realize that the core of my practice will always be my focus on families because of my personal experiences.

I continue to struggle with intermittent bouts of depression in a health care environment determined to pretend that health care providers are immune to stress. Overwork, administrative headaches, and fiscal cutbacks all contribute to depression in health care professionals. The most realistic depiction is described in The Unquiet Mind by Kay Redfield Jamison, MD. For me, though, the best medicine is the children. Welcoming a new baby into the world, while teaching the parents how to better care for her special needs is a wonder. Performing a well-child check up on a child who was not predicted to live, and who is enjoying life in their own small way, is miraculous. Discharging 21-year-old adults with disabilities from pediatric care to adult services is bitter-sweet; although I will miss them, I am proud of the potential that they have tapped and the future they have found despite all odds. Now my goal is not to be there as long as they need me, but to work myself out of a job!

My life experiences have shaped me as a nurse. My own struggles with depression have helped me provide support for struggling parents. All of these diverse ingredients have come together in one resilient pediatric nurse practitioner. My future as a nurse extends before me. Which path will I follow? I could venture into research, education, or politics, helping more children every day. In my practice, I can touch many families one at a time, and allow them to touch me. Nursing is my vocation, my mission, my service, and my profession. From nursing, I receive inspiration, motivation, validation, and strength.

CHAPTER 98

MY CHOICE

BY MARY C. MCCARTHY

From time to time I hear nurses say, "if I had it to do all over I would not go into nursing." To that, my usual response is, "If your heart is not in it, you would be better off finding a new career as soon as possible." My answer is not a cavalier or thoughtless response because I too have had occasional thoughts about my career choice ever since I made it. To decide to become a nurse was not easy or logical for me. As the daughter, granddaughter, and niece of nurses, I was well aware of the hours, conditions, and challenges of being a nurse. Although I admired the work of nurses, I did not think that it was for me.

Both of my grandmothers graduated from nursing programs during the 1920s and worked in the nursing realities of that era. One assisted a country physician in South Dakota delivering babies in small farmhouses along dusty roads. Her nursing career took a reprieve while she raised five children. She went back to nursing in a large city hospital in the 1950s. She cared for patients with polio who were often placed in iron lungs. She told fascinating stories about the nursing care given to people of all ages, backgrounds, races, and creeds.

My mother, my grandmother's oldest child, followed in her mother's footsteps. The fast pace of emergency and medical-surgical nursing sustained her through a forty year nursing career. She worked in a variety of patient care and nursing administrative areas and shifts. My mother served as a mentor for many nurses who sought advanced education, involvement in professional associations, and nursing input on health policy. An underlying belief that my mother stressed in her nursing roles was the difference that nursing care makes in a patient's experience. Nurses can help make a situation better or worse for a patient and family, and she always stressed the positive difference that a nurse can make.

My grandmother and mother were not the only people who stood as nursing role models for me. Many of the women that I knew were nurses—often friends or associates of my mother or grandmother. During my sophomore year in college, as an undeclared major, I began to notice the women whom I respected were nurses who had several common characteristics. These characteristics were a positive view on life and of nursing, a strong personal commitment to patients, an inquiring mind, an ability to balance personal and professional responsibilities, a sense of humor, and an attitude of hope.

Additionally, each woman was able to support herself and her family. The scope of nursing that presented itself to me was varied. There were nurse friends who worked in addictions/recovery, the operating room, ICU, obstetrics, public health, and nursing education. Thus, when I did decide to become a third generation nurse, I knew what I was getting into. It was a field that offered daily learning opportunities, rich opportunities for helping relationships, self-determination, and a diverse practice arena.

Now that I am approaching 50, I think about how I am promoting nursing as a career. Do I project the characteristics that I found admirable some thirty years ago? Do I talk to people about the opportunities of nursing versus the problems of nursing? Is my heart still blending the art and science of nursing? These are questions that I pose to myself. I know that I would like to leave a legacy of at least one nurse to replace me.

CHAPTER 99

A NOVICE ARMY NURSE MAKES A DIFFERENCE

BY PIA LABIO INGUITO

After having graduated with my BSN from the University of Southern California and getting commissioned in the Army Nurse Corps in 1989, my first duty assignment as a second lieutenant was at Brooke Army Medical Center (BAMC)—Beach Pavilion, Ward 42B-Cardiothoracic Surgery, where I primarily took care of coronary artery bypass graft patients. During my two years there, I gained vast clinical experience assisting with code blues, reading and interpreting cardiac rhythms, starting IVs, and caring for chest-leg incisions. The most rewarding moments for me were the interactions I had with my patients helping them with their immediate needs—bathing, dressing, pain control, and walking after major procedures. Just being there to actively listen to them when they needed to express their thoughts and emotions about the ordeal was rewarding.

I thought my four years would be spent working with cardiac patients, but instead, I received orders to transfer to Ward 43C—Orthopedic Surgery in the early 1990s when the Gulf War was starting. During this difficult time, my duties as a soldier and as an army nurse came first. My clinical experiences expanded as I cared for young soldiers who returned with orthopedic trauma injuries from Desert Storm.

One day while I was on duty, I checked my mailbox and to my surprise, I received an unexpected letter from one of the heart patients that I had cared for during my days on Ward 42B. Of all the recognitions and awards I have received for my work as a nurse, this letter has made the greatest impact on me.

LT Pia Labio,

I remembered how great you were to me during my 5X bypass in Jan '90 so I chased you down and you're on nights! Sorry, I missed you. I've decided to go to nursing school when I retire in Dec. this year because of you. I hope you remember me—CW3 (then I was "2") Dan Madison. I had to come here for a stress test. No problem! I run 4 miles daily.

Love n' Luck!

Dan Madison

Throughout these years, I have kept this letter to remind me that being a nurse can make a difference in someone's life in ways one cannot always see or comprehend. As a novice army nurse, I was just doing what I was taught to do and doing it to the best of my ability. With the many rewarding nursing experiences I have had since my days in the Army Nurse Corps, I always remember to lead by example. You never know who will follow!

CHAPTER 100

ANGELS OF MERCY

BY MICHELE N. PEDULLA

As long as I can remember, I wanted to take care of people. At first I thought that I'd be a doctor, but soon realized that a nurse was a better fit for me. I completed my Bachelors of Science in Nursing, and started my clinical practice on a pediatric hematology-oncology floor. I continued to work in this specialty for 18 years, touching many lives, and being equally touched by their lives. It has been almost a symbiotic relationship, one in which I give patients and their families strength and assistance during difficult times. In return, I am blessed with the experiences of miracle cures or of witnessing passages into the next life. I was blessed with two beautiful daughters and a loving husband. All of my loved ones have grown up on my stories of faith, strength, love, and self-lessness.

I thought that I had a good handle on it all. Then, my father became ill. He was ill for a long time, and his quality of life was minimal. As I realized that he was nearing death, it became very difficult for me. As a nurse, I knew the signs and knew what needed to be done to help my father pass as comfortably as possible. We moved him to a private room, so that the family could be together. You see, I come from a family of eleven children. So all of us spent the night with him, laughing, talking, crying, and cherishing the last moments with him. The new graduate nurse who was assigned to my father cried, and I found myself comforting her, because I had been through this so many times before.

I worked hard in the two years to come, remembering my dad. I worked on fulfilling my lifelong dream of becoming a nurse practitioner. My father passed on at the beginning of my first semester. I knew that he would want me to continue, so I worked hard with the support of my husband, my family, and my friends.

As I approached my final semester, I felt great! I thought of how proud my father would have been. I spoke to my mom often, and she was so supportive of me. Then, I received an e-mail from my brother. My mother, who had raised 11 children, still taught full-time, remembered every birthday, anniversary, and made each of her 30 grandchildren feel special, just wasn't herself. He wrote that she was hardly eating and had not been able to walk up the stairs to her bed for a few weeks. She had been able to teach every day, but would come home and take a nap. When I saw her a month ago, she seemed fine, but then again, she was always good at covering up anything that had to do with her own discomfort.

I was to go to work that morning, but had an overwhelming need to see her. After dropping off the girls at school, I drove two hours to surprise her at school. You see, if I called her and said that I was coming, she would have assured me that she was fine. I surprised her, and she looked so relieved. After school, she came home and napped. She had made an appointment to see the doctor early the next morning, only after she was assured that she could get to school to teach. We went together, and I returned to work that night. The next day, she was admitted to the hospital, a place that she hadn't been in 35 years, when she gave birth to my youngest brother!

Thinking about how much she feared hospitals, physicians, and feeling ill, I knew that I, the nurse, needed to be with her. I went to the hospital the next day, and spent the next 12 days with her. This was the most eye-opening experience I'd ever had as a nurse. As I accompanied her for every test, every meeting with a specialist or new nurse that came to see her, I felt that I had to protect her. Here was a 74-year-old lady lying in bed. I grew exhausted explaining that she had not been ill, she was a vibrant lady, and she had been teaching up until the day she was admitted. Flowers were delivered in abundance. Cards from the students and loved ones covered the walls. As a nurse, I knew what the test results meant. As a daughter, I didn't want to know. As a pediatric nurse for so many years, I had become quite comfortable with my knowledge level. As a daughter, I looked for angels of mercy to help us through this time.

Our angels of mercy came through! They were the staff nurses at the hospital. Some had only months of experience while others had decades. They all had a common thread—they were among those of us who followed the calling of helping others throughout their lives. Ruth Ann had a calming, soothing way of helping my mom. Jen assisted the family by joining in the laughter and the tears. Denise, with her strong faith, calmed us all. Patrika, with her kind, gentle words, helped Mom through the nights. Then, when I felt that I could not handle any more, Ellen came to our rescue. She knew Mom personally, and came to help in any way she could. She listened, she counseled, and she moved mountains. She was there when the surgeons came out and said that there was nothing to do but take her home. Ellen pulled her bureaucratic strings and helped move things along so that we could have Mom home. Hospice came in, respected our privacy, and gave us literature, strength, and the reassurance that we were all doing everything right. Seventeen days after that first visit to the doctor and six days after surgery, my mother died. Watching my mom take her last breath, with all of her children close by, many sleeping, I once again thanked God that I was a nurse, and that I had the strength, the knowledge, and the support of all my fellow angels of mercy to allow my mom to experience a high quality of life and death.

I was able to return to teaching, work, and everyday life. As a nurse, I will never be the same. I wear my guardian angel pin to work to remind me of the other side—the struggles and pain that families experience. I thank God for all the angels of mercy that have helped my loved ones and me. Wherever I go, I vow to continue to work on being someone's angel of mercy.

Contributor Biographies

Shelley B. Adams, RN, BSN graduated in 1980 from Northeast Louisiana University in Monroe, Louisiana. She married an Army flight student after graduation and has lived in many locations throughout the United States. Shelley is currently a Director of Nursing and Clinical Services in a psychiatric hospital. She will complete her Masters of Science in Nursing in 2005. She and her husband have three children, one grandchild, and a beloved Basenji named Kesia.

Wendell Alderson, RN, was born and raised in northern California, which has been his home, except for three years in Saudi Arabia. His specialty is emergency nursing in intensive care units and medivac helicopters. Currently Wendell works in a recovery room. He and his partner enjoy traveling and bike riding. Cooking and working in his yard are therapeutic after a hard day's work.

Melody C. Antoon, RN, MSN lives in Southeast Texas with her daughters. She teaches at local university. She has two baccalaureate degrees, one in Environmental Health and the other in Nursing. She earned a Master's Degree in Nursing from the University of Southeastern Louisiana in Baton Rouge. After several years of hospital nursing, Melody began working in home health where she stayed for many years. Her career is now focused on teaching.

Theresa Bagenski, LPN, grew up in Connecticut. After high school, she married and moved to London, England, where her first child was born. They returned to Connecticut. Theresa went to the Morse School of Nursing after her children were grown up. She loves to paint with oils and her life-long ambition is to sing God Bless America in front of a large crowd, just like Kate Smith.

Kathy Grimley Baker, RN, NP, MS is a fourth generation San Franciscan. She graduated from the University of San Francisco and began her career at Stanford University Medical Center. Ten years ago, Kathy became a part-time faculty member at the University. Now, she works part-time at Stanford and has the joy of seeing the progress of her formed students. She thinks nursing is the best job in the world.

Amy Barnes, RN, BSN, MA has been a registered nurse for 27 years. She has worked in the hospital setting as a staff nurse and educator. For the past seven years, she has been in school health. Currently, Amy is a Health Specialist for

Head Start. She is married with two grown children and a very spoiled Jack Russell terrier. Her interests include cycling and antiquing.

Amy Blanchard, RN, BSN is a 2001 graduate of the University of Vermont, School of Nursing. She is a lieutenant in the Army. Amy is in the 28th Combat Support Hospital in Operation Iraqi Freedom.

Margaret Bonen, BS, RN, C, has been a Registered Nurse since 1986, is certified in Psychiatric Mental Health and has a Bachelors of Science in Health Arts. She has worked in General Surgery, Adult and Adolescent Drug and Alcohol in-patient rehabilitation, Adolescent Psychiatric in-patient treatment, Psychiatric Home Health, Step-down Open Heart/Cardiac Critical Care, Manager Dementia/Alzheimer's, and is currently an Assistant Director of Nursing in long-term care. A member of the American Nurses Association and Indiana State Nurses Association since 1985, she was also a past active member of the Indiana Peer Review for impaired nurses through the Indiana State Nurses Association. Episcopalian, her father is a retired Episcopal Bishop of Northern Indiana, and her mother is a retired English teacher. One of five children herself, she is the mother of two grown children and has four grandchildren. She is recently widowed.

Susan Grady Bristol, RN has been a nurse for 26 years. She is currently a pediatric office nurse. She is also a freelance writer who has been published in numerous health journals as well as popular publications such as *Family Fun* magazine and *Chicken Soup for the Soul*. Susan is the mother of three sons and makes her home in Omaha, Nebraska with her husband Dennis.

Steven L. Brown, LCDR, NC, USN, graduated from the University of Toledo in 1992. Immediately after graduation, he received his commission in the United States Navy as an Ensign. Since that time, he has been stationed in the United States and in Italy. Currently, Steven is the nurse manager of the Intensive Care Unit and Medical-Surgical Units in Pensacola, Florida. He is married with four children.

JoAnn Brakora Bugbee, RN, BC, is the Nursing Staff Development Coordinator at State Hospital South, on the two state psychiatric hospitals in Idaho. She has pursued various nursing specialty areas across the country. Jo Ann has held leadership roles in professional organizations and has received awards for achievement and leadership where she has worked. Jo Ann plays the organ in local community churches. She is a grandmother.

Peggy S. Campbell, RN, BSN, began her nursing career as a licensed practical nurse in order to support her family. With colleagues, she planned and implemented one of the first hospital-based ground transportation systems. Peggy developed standards and protocols for city regulations and ambulance certification. She is active on her community planning board. Her poetry has won awards. She has a consulting business for senior citizens.

Denise Casaubon, RN, BS, has been a nurse for over 10 years. She loves being a nurse because she gets to interact with all types of people in a variety of situations. Many times the situations are stressful. Denise travels around the country as a consultant to health care facilities.